APHASIA INSIDE OUT

APHASIA INSIDE OUT

Reflections on Communication Disability

Edited by
Susie Parr, Judy Duchan *and* **Carole Pound**

Open University Press

Open University Press
McGraw-Hill Education
McGraw-Hill House
Shoppenhangers Road
Maidenhead
Berkshire
England
SL6 2QL

email: enquiries@openup.co.uk
world wide web: www.openup.co.uk

First published 2003

A catalogue record of this book is available from the British Library

ISBN 0 335 21144 5 (pb) 0 335 21145 3 (hb)

Library of Congress Cataloging-in-Publication Data
CIP data has been applied for

Typeset by RefineCatch Limited, Bungay, Suffolk
Printed in the UK by Bell & Bain Ltd, Glasgow

Contents

List of figures and tables

Notes on contributors

Maria Black is a clinical linguist in the Department of Human Communication Science, University College London. She has written on language, language processing, aphasia and the politics of language.

Sue Boazman works as a volunteer counsellor at Connect, the communication disability network, in London. She also contributes to the development and running of counselling skills workshops at Connect. Sue has personal experience of stroke and aphasia. She is an advocate of creative therapy in her counselling and teaching and is keen to promote the use of new ways of counselling in the wider counselling arena.

Sally Byng has worked as a speech and language therapist and in higher education. She is now Chief Executive and Director of Research at Connect in London. Through her collaborations over the years in organizational development work, research and teaching she has sought to influence the content and delivery of services that are provided to people living with aphasia.

Harry Clarke trained as a counsellor following his own experience of stroke and aphasia and was awarded an Advanced Diploma at London University in 1995. Shortly afterwards he began providing a counselling service for people with aphasia and has worked at Connect since its inception.

John Clarke and Monica Clarke. John Clarke died in 2003. 'His loss of words was a double blow because he had been a psychotherapist before his stroke. His words had been his main healing tool,' says Monica, his widow. Monica lives in London where she continues Pictures Speak, the project which she and John started together, running training programmes for health and social care workers to enable them to support communication.

Judy Duchan is Professor Emerita from the State University of New York at Buffalo. She worked as a speech and language therapist in public schools in the US before becoming a clinical researcher. She is now exploring and developing ways to include those with communication disabilities in their communities.

Roberta J. Elman is President/Founder of the Aphasia Center of California. She has more than 20 years of experience working with people with communication disorders. Roberta has authored and edited numerous publications with an emphasis on group treatment. She is an American Speech and Hearing Association (ASHA) fellow and is active in the Academy of Neurologic Communication Disorders and Sciences.

Alan Hewitt is the Working Together Co-ordinator at Connect, the communication disability network, involving people with aphasia at all levels. He is Secretary of Aphasia Nottingham, a self-help group. Before he had a brain haemorrhage and aphasia in 1992, he was Head of Development at National Energy Action, a fuel poverty charity.

Chris Ireland has been a teacher, a social scientist and a counsellor. She has embarked on a new career as a poet, trainer and aphasia counsellor. Chris has written on language in education and social exclusion, counselling, aphasia and language disability.

Aura Kagan is Program, Research and Education Director at the Aphasia Institute (incorporating the Pat Arato Aphasia Centre) – an agency in Toronto, Canada, dedicated to service, awareness, education, research and advocacy for people affected by aphasia. She was instrumental in the development of Supported Conversation for Adults with Aphasia™ – a tool for increasing communicative access to life participation.

Jasvinder Khosa worked as a deputy headteacher before having a stroke in 1992. Since then he has worked as a classroom assistant, among other roles in education. Experiencing aphasia led him to an interest in the 'intrapsychic conflicts' of an individual and he is training to become an integrative psychotherapist.

Turid de Mare trained as a psychotherapeutic counsellor and worked with individuals and groups in the mental health charity MIND and in her own practice. She had a stroke in 1999 and has aphasia. She spends some of her time now at Connect, contributing to service development and education, as well as participating in many of the groups.

Becky Moss is interested in how health issues are explained to patients and consumers, and what influences how patients understand and interpret information from experts. She has worked on a communication skills programme for cancer specialists and studied the consultations of general practitioners whose patients speak limited English.

Susie Parr is Research Fellow with Connect, the communication disability network, and City University, London. Her research interests include the impact of aphasia, communication impairment and social exclusion, illness and personal narratives in aphasia, the potential of information technologies, and the application of qualitative methodologies.

Kevin Paterson is a researcher in the School of Law and Social Sciences at Glasgow Caledonian University. His research interests span the fields of disability studies and sociology of the body. He has published in various edited collections and the journal *Disability and Society*.

Tom Penman has worked as a speech and language therapist since 1986, and became London Centre Director for Connect, the communication disability network, in 2000. He has a particular interest in the development of therapies for living with aphasia, and raising awareness of the issues for people with communication disability in the wider community.

Carole Pound is Director of Therapy and Education at Connect. She has worked as a speech and language therapist in hospitals, and rehabilitation and university settings. Her interests include developing therapies that address the long-term communication, identity and lifestyle issues of living with a disability, supporting others to develop communication access and working with people with aphasia to create more inclusive structures and communities.

Leanne Togher is a speech therapist. Her current research interests include examining the interactions of people with acquired brain injury in different everyday speaking situations and describing the perceptions of older Indigenous Australians of their healthcare interactions. Leanne has also developed training programmes for community agencies based on her research findings.

Foreword

This book, which is written as a collaborative effort by people with and without aphasia, is a timely contribution to the lives of people with communication impairments and to the field of disability studies. The book has a strong orientation to the social model of disability (without being constrained by it) and brings fresh insights into the particular barriers people with aphasia face. Many of these barriers are shared, to a greater or lesser extent, with other disabled people (for example, access to information, and issues around time) but communication barriers themselves have prevented people with aphasia from having a strong voice within the disabled people's movement and within research.

I first met Susie Parr and Carole Pound nearly ten years ago when they asked me to talk about the social model of disability at a conference for speech and language therapists. I was somewhat daunted by this knowing that the social model of disability had largely been formulated by people with visual and physical impairments and did not have much to say about the particular barriers people with communication impairments may face. I soon became aware, however, that Susie and Carole saw it as their mission, in full collaboration with people with aphasia, to discover where and how the social model would fit. This is reflected in their work at Connect, which features strongly in this book. Theorizing around disability is important but this book goes further by taking a strong practical orientation with many concrete suggestions and examples that can be put into practice by people with aphasia and by everyone else in society.

The experience of living with aphasia is central to all of the chapters and, as with all impairments and disabilities, illustrates a complex mix of joy, frustration, difficulty, stress, happiness, personal growth and fulfilment. The final chapter which celebrates aphasia poetry provides a wonderful example of 'disability arts' where disability is affirmed and celebrated and where erroneous ideas about disability are questioned and dispelled. There are also some very honest accounts by speech and language therapists about their work with people with aphasia and how they grew dissatisfied with the way they practised.

It is my belief that this book will become a well respected volume within the disability studies literature and that the social model of disability will be expanded and strengthened by the insights it offers. Whether or not it will influence professional workers, who tend to be steeped in a medical and individual model of disability, I am not so sure, but the book provides detailed information and insights for anyone brave enough to change their practice in a radical way.

Sally French
University of Hertfordshire

Preface

The idea for this book grew out of a series of dialogues we had with colleagues and friends in the UK and beyond. We wanted to provide an opportunity for people to write reflectively about aphasia (a language difficulty that can follow stroke). Much has been written about this topic, but usually from a scientific or academic point of view. This book offers its authors a chance to explore their reflections and perspectives, and to write about aspects of aphasia that are not normally covered in the literature. In particular, we wanted to provide authors who have aphasia with an opportunity to publish their own reflections and insights.

The logistics of developing such a project and supporting the different contributors meant that the majority of them are associated with Connect, the communication disability network, which is based in London. Our other contributors come from different parts of the UK, Canada, Australia and the US. We hope this reflects our sense that much of the thinking and practice of Connect is linked with what is going on elsewhere.

The chapters cover a wide range of topics. In Chapter 1, the introduction, the editors discuss the contributions to this book in the context of current disability theory. In Chapter 2, Jasvinder Khosa reflects on the way in which aphasia has changed his life and affected his sense of who he is. Chapter 3 sees Maria Black (who is multilingual) and Chris Ireland (who has aphasia) talking about the relationship between language and thinking from these different perspectives. Sue Boazman, in Chapter 4, discusses personal and professional changes brought about by the different consequences of her stroke. Aura Kagan, in Chapter 5, discusses the idea of community and tries to understand what this might mean for people with aphasia. In Chapter 6, Alan Hewitt and Sally Byng discuss their different routes towards collaborative work and explore the idea of social engagement. Leanne Togher also considers this issue, in Chapter 7, and explores how the power balance between therapists and people with aphasia might be changed. In Chapter 8, Harry Clarke describes his work as a counsellor in the context of his own aphasia. Tom Penman and Turid de Mare draw on their experience as users and providers of group work to reflect on the differences between aphasia therapy and psychotherapy, in Chapter 9. In Chapter 10, Roberta Elman, Susie Parr and Becky Moss consider the potential benefits of the Internet for people with aphasia, and the barriers they face in using it. In Chapter 11, Monica and John Clarke describe how communication between them was enhanced by drawing and determination. Chapter 12 sees Susie Parr, Kevin Paterson and Carole Pound discussing the ways in which time can be a barrier for people with communication difficulties. The final chapter, by Chris Ireland and Carole Pound, acts as a showcase for Chris's poetry, and her celebration of language that is different and creative.

We hope that the book will have a wide appeal. We envisage it being of interest to disability theorists, rehabilitation professionals, linguists, philosophers, those interested in creative writing, and people personally affected by aphasia. Each chapter is written in a very different style, and not all of them will appeal to everyone or be accessible to every reader. With that in mind, we have prefaced each chapter with a list of the key points, written in straightforward language. We hope this makes *Aphasia Inside Out* more accessible and enjoyable.

Finally, we would like to thank our contributors, our colleagues and all those who have made *Aphasia Inside Out* such a pleasure to work on.

Susie Parr, Judy Duchan and Carole Pound

1

Setting the scene

Susie Parr, Judy Duchan and Carole Pound

Key points

- This book is made up of a set of essays.
- About half of the authors have aphasia. The others don't.
- The authors write from many different points of view. They are counsellors, carers, teachers, therapists, linguists and people studying disability issues.
- We asked people to write about things they think are important but which don't usually get written about.
- We also wanted people to reflect: to think about their work and their lives in the context of aphasia.
- The book allows people to write in ways that are unusual or different.
- We wanted to give people with aphasia an opportunity to write about it, from the inside. Often, they don't get the chance to do this.
- We hope the book will appeal to lots of different people, including some people who are personally affected by aphasia. There are some good ideas here. Some chapters are easier to read than others.
- Others who might read the book include therapists and rehabilitation workers, and people interested in disability, language and writing.
- The authors have written about a number of different things with relation to aphasia: poetry, the Internet, identity or sense of self, community, the difficulties faced by people with aphasia, relationships in therapy, and getting involved.

- Although these topics are all different, there are a number of themes that run through the chapters:
  1 Barriers, or things that get in the way, for people with aphasia.
  2 The effect of aphasia on one's sense of self or identity.
  3 New ways of thinking and doing things.
  4 Celebrating aphasia.
- We think it's important that people know more about aphasia, particularly those in the disability movement. We hope *Aphasia Inside Out* helps this to happen.

This book contains a selection of reflective essays about aphasia (a communication impairment that commonly follows stroke affecting one's ability to use and understand spoken and written language). Half of the contributors to the book have personal experience of aphasia. Authors with and without aphasia write from the perspective of different backgrounds and disciplines including disability studies, linguistics, counselling, teaching, psychotherapy and aphasia therapy.

Aphasia Inside Out provides a platform for a group of people who hitherto have had little access to the mainstream literature concerning the relationship between disability and society. They have been silent, but this is not because they have nothing to say. Nor do they lack personal or professional expertise in discussions of disability and difference. So what is it that silences their voice?

It could be suggested that their silence is due to the nature of their impairment: aphasia brings with it a difficulty in pinning down and translating thoughts into words, trouble following densely written texts, and prevents engagement in the rapid cut and thrust of debate. But to focus on the impairment would be to overlook the role others (including disabled people) play, in either supporting or sidelining the contributions of those with communication impairments such as aphasia.

People with aphasia rarely get the opportunity to put forward their ideas, even within the 'my story' genre of lay accounts. In this volume we value the reflections of authors who have an inside knowledge of aphasia. We hope that this book will contribute to theory, philosophy and practice concerning aphasia. As such it should be stimulating and challenging to those who are affected by or concerned with aphasia, either personally or in their work.

The premise of the book is to provide an opportunity for writers to explore aspects of aphasia that are usually passed over by prevailing academic discourses. Accordingly the topics addressed in these essays are diverse and often unconventional: poetry, community, time, engagement, the Internet, confidence, counselling, identity, creativity and so on. The intention behind inviting these contributions was to offer the authors liberation from the tightly scientific or pragmatic focus of their respective disciplines, to encourage reflection and subjectivity, to foster different, collaborative and non-traditional styles of writing, and, most importantly, to provide a platform for the work of those who arguably have the most profound understanding of communication impairment.

For readers from the field of disability studies, *Aphasia Inside Out* presents some challenging insights on the nature of disabling barriers, identity issues, and the presence and impact of the impairment itself. For lay readers, including some with aphasia, many chapters offer shared experience, affirmation and ideas about recovery. Those concerned with therapy and rehabilitation will find new ideas about practice, roles and relationships. The book calls for reflection and self-scrutiny and offers some practical and creative ideas. Linguists and philosophers will gain insights into the relationship between language and identity, and those interested in creative writing will find the diverse styles of the chapters, and the ways in which they have been constructed, intriguing.

Aphasia Inside Out is grounded in the social model of disability. This model represents disability as a product of externally imposed disadvantages and social restrictions, rather than as an inevitable result of the impairment itself (Oliver and Barnes 1998). A number of the chapters are concerned with identifying and discussing some of the more subtle *disabling barriers* faced by people with aphasia.

Our book raises and addresses the controversial issue of *disabled identity* in relation to communication impairments (Reeve 2002). This is a contested topic, and the source of much conflict within the field of disability studies, partly because it distracts attention away from external barriers (Watson 2002). We focus on this issue in this book because aphasia profoundly affects language and therefore has implications for self-expression and conceptions of the self. Talking about aphasia means talking about language and changing identities. Some authors address the issue of identity by writing about transformation and affirmation, a kind of reconfiguring of the self (Reeve 2002). They propose creative personal responses to language impairment, and bring a personal dimension to the struggle for social inclusion.

In a number of chapters rehabilitation professionals, sometimes in collaboration with people who have aphasia, scrutinize their practice and reconsider their roles and their relationships. The tone of these chapters is tentative and enquiring, rather than dogmatic, as befits a cautious process of reconfiguration and realignment. Readers will find that some authors are more comfortable than others when stepping outside professional discourses.

The 'inside' of inside out can be taken to mean inside the person, or inside the impairment of aphasia. This focus on 'inside' may not, at first glance, seem to be in keeping with a social model. We feel, however, that a grounded social model needs to consider disability from within the perspectives of disabled people. Many essays in this book are therefore concerned with the relationship between impairment and disability. We focus on understanding and acknowledging the experience of the disability as well as identifying and dismantling disabling barriers. This relationship between impairment and disability is relatively unexplored both in disability studies and aphasia therapy. We therefore hope to offer new opportunities for investigation and theory building.

Why 'inside out'?

The term 'inside out' concerns the external expression of internal feelings, beliefs and musings. Our authors, writing both from inside and outside the experience of aphasia, were encouraged to explore new lines of thinking as they reflected on the life implications of language difference and language loss. Jasvinder Khosa describes his nuanced and different identities in relation to the different languages he speaks and how his aphasia altered his linguistic and cultural identities. Maria Black and Chris Ireland dialogue with one another about mismatches between language and thinking, and how these mismatches increased for each of them. In Chris's case these increased when she had a stroke resulting in aphasia and for Maria, when she shifted from languages that she was well grounded in, to new ones.

Another meaning of 'inside out' has to do with feelings of social exclusion resulting from aphasia. Those with aphasia are left out, non-members, ostracized, marginalized. Aura Kagan discusses this by stressing the need for multiple 'communities' (with a small 'c') to be restored as part of the everyday lives of those with aphasia. Alan Hewitt and Sally Byng explore forms of partnership, and in tracing their own professional and personal experience argue for the importance of 'engagement' in achieving an authentic sense of self-fulfilment. Susie Parr, Kevin Paterson and Carole Pound explore the many ways that disabled people are excluded because of the time requirements of everyday life. And Roberta Elman, Susie Parr and Becky Moss describe the many barriers that those with impairments meet when accessing the Internet. They go on to offer some suggestions for how these barriers might be reduced.

A third way that 'inside out' figures in this volume is reflected in a set of essays concerning how to support those with aphasia as they develop internal ways of managing new or changing identities. The business of helping people 'adjust' or 'cope' is often taken as an impairment-based approach with a focus on changing the disabled person rather than on social or physical barriers. The authors in this book suggest that these fixed role definitions and views of counselling and therapy be reworked.

They recommend that disabled people take a more active role in therapy processes and that the focus of the therapy be widened to include life circumstances and external barriers, as well as inner change. These two shifts, towards empowerment and the dismantling of disabling barriers, reframes counselling to be more in keeping with a social model of disability.

Tom Penman and Turid de Mare talk about different professional ways of approaching group work. They advocate that therapists, whatever their ilk, become facilitators rather than leaders of groups and that members of aphasia therapy groups have responsibility for what transpires. Harry Clarke, a counsellor with aphasia, also argues for a less dominant role for therapists of people with aphasia – they should talk less and listen more! Sue Boazman reflects on her own experiences first as a manager, then as a person recovering from aphasia and now as a counsellor. She invites us to consider recovery from aphasia as a series of ups and downs in confidence and sense of control based on the interrelationships of impairments and life circumstances.

Another way that 'inside out' is used in this book relates to supporting people with aphasia in expressing themselves. This struggle to get the inside thoughts out can be viewed from an impairment perspective as a difficulty the person has with language, or from a disability perspective as a poverty of ways that those interacting with people with aphasia have in supporting their expression. Monica Clarke in a lively depiction of her conversations with her husband, John, who had severe aphasia, shows how successful communication can be achieved, given creativity, flexibility, persistence and the right resources. And Leanne Togher gives insight into traditional ways of thinking by aphasia therapists, arguing for a more conversationally based approach in which client and therapist share meaningful experiences – ones that they can talk about later. Finally, the chapter by Chris Ireland and Carole Pound offers a powerful way of making language expression available to those with aphasia – through celebrating language differences and seeing them in terms of poetic licence and legitimate expression rather than as 'language errors'.

Aphasia and access

A major issue that arose in the course of putting this book together concerned access. We first conceived of the book as a way to create a publication venue for those with aphasia, who have little access to expressing to others their personal and professional concerns. This lack of access is particularly true in a publishing world that emphasizes professional discourse written in an academic style. Those with the authority to generate and edit a volume such as this one generally approach established authors who are familiar with such discourses and, of course, at ease with language. Part of the editing process involves discussion and debate with the contributors, drawing on these shared resources.

In editing *Aphasia Inside Out* we were not always able to draw from those familiar with writing and publishing. This led to a need for us to provide support for some of our authors, giving verbal shape to their reflections for the purposes of publication. In that way we were able to draw on the expertise of the insiders who live the challenge of language impairment, and to have them join a discourse that has not only excluded them but has also been conducted in a language that seems foreign.

We also became aware when debating possible audiences for the book that speech/language therapists and other professionals working in the field of aphasia have had little access to the literature in the disability studies. Similarly those in disability studies have little exposure to professional writings in the field of aphasia. This is not unusual. Members of one discipline seldom explore outside their area because of time and informational barriers. Typically, those inside a discipline write for their peers, using technical jargon, presupposing common backgrounds and excluding the uninitiated.

Cross-disciplinary barriers have been exacerbated by the disability lobby's critique of rehabilitation specialists. Those in the disability movement have complained about professionals' unreflective exercising of power and their undue focus on impairments at the expense of meeting the social challenges of exclusion. Some have called this the 'tyranny of professional discourses' (Gillman *et al.* 1997).

While sharing many of the concerns voiced by the disability movement, we have sought in this book to encourage rehabilitation professionals to consider the implications of the social model.

Another major issue associated with access has to do with those with aphasia engaging with the disabled people's movement. The disabled people's movement does not represent the entire range of people with impairments (Shakespeare 1993). This is certainly the case for people with aphasia who have had virtually no voice and no presence in this context.

This is a particularly challenging aspect of access, since aphasia is an impairment that affects language: the most powerful weapon in the armoury of the disabled people's movement. Aphasia compromises a person's ability to talk and write, and read and understand. Sharing and expressing ideas, and listening to others are critical functions in the process of mobilizing and politicizing a minority and bringing about change. When language is compromised by an impairment such as aphasia, negotiation, campaigning, education, debate and argument become difficult, if not impossible. For these reasons, people who struggle to communicate are often sidelined by a movement which should be representing them, championing their cause and sharing authority. We feel this need not be the case and our authors offer an example of how these access issues can be surmounted.

Finally, this book is concerned with access for those with communication differences. The writing of Chris Ireland in this volume not only requires courage on the part of the author in challenging language standards and breaking rules, but on the part of publishers in opening up a strikingly different linguistic landscape. We seldom see texts that are not 'cleaned up' by spellcheckers and proofreaders. Writing, with the possible exception of poetry and creative writing, is not a medium that readily promotes language difference or communication access for all.

So, much of this book is concerned with gaining access. It offers a venue and support for the writing of people with aphasia. It provides accessible ideas to those in disability studies and aphasia therapy, calling for a common discourse. It suggests that a focus on the specific nature of the impairment, in a volume based in the social model, can make those with aphasia a more visible and powerful presence within the disability movement.

Power and authority, discomfort and clarity

The process of preparing this volume for publication has been challenging, bringing discomfort and concern along with clarity and communication. As editors we have the power to invite, select, commission and focus the collection, and to support the development of individual contributions. We are also in the position to exclude those with an interest in aphasia who are not known, are not able to write or who require what seems an unworkable level of support. As the process unfolds, while setting our sights on egalitarian, inclusionary practices, we are forced to exercise our power and our privilege.

Struggles with identity, culture, role and expertise also emerge from the stories of our contributors. While some essays rest on a more confident foundation, a level of discomfort is evident in their questioning of their position and expertise. In some instances this questioning forms the content of their contribution (Hewitt and Byng; Togher) whereas in others the discomfort emerges more subtly as they talk about different styles and dominant voices (Penman and de Mare; Black and Ireland; Ireland and Pound). Jasvinder Khosa writes about how conflicts between different cultural aspects of his identity developed during his childhood and have been consolidated by his experience of aphasia.

Difficulties with the process of collaborative writing are addressed explicitly in some contributions (Ireland and Pound). Themes of power, authority, dominant and vanishing voices, constraining or emancipatory language have criss-crossed the production phases of this volume, prompting different moments of insight and discomfort for all. For example, in supporting people with aphasia to catch hold of opaque, cellophane wrapped ideas (Khosa), a communication supporter might justifiably offer structures, concepts and words to help the storyteller fix on a means of expression. Yet words both shape and constrain meaning, possibly adding a colour, an emphasis, a nuance that was not a part of the original thought.

People with aphasia require language and confidence to challenge and question those supporting them. When time and energy are limited, the temptation is to accept fast-track 'solutions' of suggested words and questions, to defer to those with professional or academic status and style of expression, and to underplay personal expression.

Negotiating roles in writing and editing

Negotiations between authors, co-authors and editors took different forms depending upon the individuals, their roles and the tasks at hand. The role of 'communication supporter' (for authors with and without aphasia) has covered diverse tasks including:

- interviewing, questioning to clarify, extend and articulate ideas, checking meaning and word selection;
- listening, bearing witness to personal accounts, supporting the narrative telling of stories;
- recording, note-taking, supporting memory for themes and thoughts;
- acting as reflector, sounding board, mirror for thoughts, words and nuances;
- producing first drafts, suggesting structures and 'translations', meeting to check interpretations and translations, highlighting unclear passages, expanding first ideas;
- word processing, proofreading, checking references for accuracy;
- motivating, encouraging, supporting people to reach for an extra level of clarity while being sensitive to the linguistic demands of yet another struggle for words.

As well as writing, contributors and editors were acting as conversation and narrative partners and administrative assistants, all of which raised different issues concerning authorship and privilege.

The authors and editors of this book have struggled to find the language to reveal the inside worlds of self-reflection and personal experience. We hope that the essays in the volume will lead to an on-going exploration of communication styles, personal and professional identities, and different approaches to collaboration and engagement. While many of the themes of this book will be familiar, we suggest that the issue of the communicative competence and style – of people both with and without a language impairment – poses an additional obstacle to breaching the power divide. Communicating clearly while negotiating communication difference is an exciting new challenge.

References

Gillman, M., Swain, J. and Heyman, B. (1997) Life history or 'case' history: the objectification of people with learning difficulties through the tyranny of professional discourses, *Disability and Society*, 12: 675–94.

Oliver, M. and Barnes, C. (1998) *Disabled People and Social Policy: From Exclusion to Inclusion*. Harlow: Addison Wesley Longman.

Reeve, D. (2002) Negotiating psycho-emotional dimensions of disability and their influence on identity constructions, *Disability and Society*, 17(5): 493–508.

Shakespeare, T. (1993) Disabled peoples' self organisation: a new social movement? *Disability, Handicap and Society*, 8: 249–64.

Watson, N. (2002) Well I know this is going to sound very strange to you, but I don't see myself as a disabled person: identity and disability, *Disability and Society*, 17(5): 509–27.

2

Still life of a chameleon: aphasia and its impact on identity

Jasvinder Khosa

Key points

- Jasvinder tells the story of his stroke and its impact on his life.
- He looks back at his childhood and youth and talks about the many changes he experienced when he was younger, for example, moving between India and Northern Ireland and living with different members of his family.
- Each time he found himself in new circumstances he tried to fit in, for example, by switching between Panjabi and English, and by using different accents in different situations and with different people.
- Changes after his stroke meant that Jasvinder lost his ability to speak and understand Panjabi with ease, to use language for humour and to be quick with words.
- He also talks about the changes in his family relationships, his work and his career after his stroke.
- Aphasia has made Jasvinder question who he is and how his identity is evolving.
- He feels exhilarated, but at the same time he sometimes feels lost.
- He talks about the benefits and insights that aphasia has brought him, like allowing him to 'just be'.

Bechara samjada nehi – bas damakh firgaiya. Pichley janam deh karm bhughat neh pendah hai. (Poor man, he can't understand – mind has gone crazy. That's our [the family's] karma. It is punishment from the previous life.)

This is my mum, Bibbiji, crying out between her wails. Bibbiji had arrived from India when she heard about my stroke and had come to stay with me in my house in Bingley, West Yorkshire. She had come to see me, of course, and to give a break to my then wife, Jill, from nursing me, a few weeks after I had come out of hospital. I was almost mute and in a wheelchair, paralysed on my right-hand side, and had facial palsy. Bibbiji was shocked to see me in this state and broke down. I, in turn, started to worry about her ability to care for herself and my wife, as she spoke little English. This led to me suffering my first major epileptic seizure a day after her arrival. I went back to the hospital and my consultant advised the family to leave me alone to convalesce, and guard me from any kind of emotional disturbance. After a few weeks visiting other relatives, Bibbiji went back to India. God knows what she went through, emotionally.

In February 1997 I went to Punjab, India, five years after the brain haemorrhage to a family wedding and the first time that I had gone back 'home' since my dad's death there in 1993. It was a visit with strong emotional and psychological contrasts. My memory of that visit is tied together by the wedding photos and little else. In hindsight it told me how much I had and have missed and this in large part due the 'loss' of my Panjabi.

In this chapter I want to explain how aphasia has led me to address my identity issue, by understanding the implications of being severely limited in using my mother tongue. Aphasia has not just been a disadvantage. In hindsight, the brain haemorrhage and subsequent aphasia has forced me to gather the flotsam and jetsam of my life and do some spring cleaning: throwing the rubbish away that I had gathered over the years that was no longer useful and keeping the bits that are precious. I am grateful for the opportunity that writing this has given me to go through a process that led me to an unexpected, and perhaps, an inevitable outcome.

Although this is my unique experience, I hope it can be of benefit to others, who may have had a similar experience which among other things led to a change in identity. I also hope that the chapter can benefit clinicians serving clients who are bilingual or multilingual.

In March 1992 I suffered a brain haemorrhage in the Lake District where I was holidaying with my ex-wife. I ended up at Newcastle General Hospital. My first memory is waking up from my coma after the first brain operation to the sound of my sister, in her Northern Ireland accent reading *Japji Sahab* – morning Sikh prayers – by my bedside. Although my Panjabi was not ever developed enough to understand sacred concepts, I felt secure when I heard the familiar cadences, intonations and rhythms of my mother tongue. I cannot recall for certain, but I have the suspicion that I recognized (or understood) only Panjabi when it was spoken for the first few hours and days I was conscious in hospital. Together with the Geordie accent of the nurses, which is musically similar to the Irish accent,

I first thought I was in Ireland, the country where I grew up and where some of my family still resides. I imagined I was in Derry, in the hospital where I had spent time as a child with asthma. It was rather like being born again.

When I was well enough, I was transferred to the hospital in Bradford, from Newcastle, where I had surgery. Although I was told that I would never walk or talk again, I was provided with a (very good) speech therapist to reclaim my English. I had therapy for over two years. In the process I largely lost my Irish accent and acquired a 'foreign accent syndrome', like some people who have aphasia when learning to speak. I had no therapy in Panjabi – the only speech therapy in my mother tongue was practice with the Panjabi-speaking family in Birmingham who were cousins, their elders, their children, and later in India. I had occasional encounters with other Panjabi friends in Bradford who spoke a different form of the language than I did, Mirpuri Punjabi in Pakistan. My English is now fairly well developed, and is developing, while my Panjabi is woefully inadequate.

'You speak like a white person' my relatives have told me on a number of occasions when my sisters, both of whom had married 'out' in other words, they did not have an arranged marriage, were not in earshot. This was not aimed just at my ideas, which are alien to them, but at the broken, extremely hesitant Panjabi I now speak, with an accent of a Colonel Blimp figure in the British Raj films. Therapy only in English, meant my tongue and mouth had difficulty moving in any other way.

Of course the difficulty has not been just confined to my own speech, but also to understanding of language that others – my mother and other relatives – speak to me. I do not have the stamina to follow conversations. After a few minutes my ears, my mind, are exhausted. Rather like a radio struggling to tune in to long-wave radio signals in an another shore and have a piercing high-pitched sound that says; 'Danger! Overload. Switch off.' I cannot keep pace; I'm off stage, not where the action is; I have been relegated down to the audience. So, at times, I'm very much an onlooker, not a player.

Let me say from the outset that my memory in respect to language has been damaged, so words or phrases often are lost unless I write them down or talk to someone soon after the event. If I don't do either of these – the feeling, the atmosphere is preserved somehow, and it comes out to the surface when something similar happens. I say to myself 'this has happened before' (a kind of reality déjà vu) and still cannot remember the event unless prompted. Usually, I have no memory of the exact words. What is more, I often have a problem with chronology, the sequence of events as they occurred. This same process is what happens after I have read something or watched a movie. This is true for both languages. But my verbal memory is much better in the second language than it is for my mother tongue.

I've got a complicated family history and this led to an equally complicated relationship with my language and identity. I had for a long time a disjointed view of it. After my stroke I wanted to change my identity for a number of reasons. Until my stroke I was a successful professional in the field of education. Privately I was known for being funny and quick witted. In the course of my life, like everyone, I had also done things which I was not proud of. I felt that with aphasia I had the opportunity to make a clean break with everything in my past which I did not like, and also give myself a break from the expectations I felt people might have of me: I had lost my linguistic power. I was disabled and epileptic. I was treated differently. I acquired a new role, that of the listener and observer. I felt different. I decided to make a break from the old to the new – a familiar experience for me.

I have at least two identities and two first names to match. Up until my stroke, I was known as Binday, by family and friends. Bibbiji named me Balvinder. Binday is a short informal version of Balvinder. The Sikh rituals for naming were not observed, however. Some days later, my father, Pitaji, feeling uncomfortable about it, chose a new name for me: Jasvinder. This is the name on my birth certificate. However, nobody called me Jasvinder. I was still known to everyone, my family, my friends, my colleagues, by the name of Binday.

After the stroke something changed. I wanted to be called by my real official name: Jasvinder. I had a little ceremony and told my friends to call me by my official name. An Irish friend of mine celebrated this in a poem, which I have stuck on my kitchen wall: 'Today is Bin-Day'.

I was born and brought up in the North of Ireland in a Sikh Panjabi family, youngest of six. Prior to my brain haemorrhage in 1992, the accent and vernacular of the region of my birth was still very much discernible in my speech (not just speech but language). I remember my childhood as a constant uprooting from one community to another, from one country to another, from one language to another, from one accent to another. Perhaps as a result, I have acquired chameleon-like skills to adjust to different environments.

My parents had always planned to return to India once they had made 'enough' money in Ireland. They feared also that they might be sent back to India, if British policies changed. Enoch Powell's 'Rivers of blood' speech in 1968 confirmed my parents' fear. My mother saved for this and left us early on, when I was two years old, to buy a few acres of land in Punjab, where we planned to return. We attempted to go back twice. Each time, it was to be for good. Each time I had to resign myself to the loss of a life and the start of another.

The first time I went back to India was in 1967 via Birmingham where

Pitaji got a job working in a foundry for six months. I was 6 years old. Pitaji took three children back to live in Punjab with the intention of living there for good. My older siblings, for various reasons, stayed behind. My sister, brother and I started to learn Panjabi. However, very quickly our health deteriorated, partly because we had gone during the hottest time of year in June. We suffered heat rash, diarrhoea, general stomach problems and malaria. We had to go back to Britain with Pitaji, because the funds had run dry after two years. Bibbiji had to stay behind to look after the farm, a sad and forlorn figure.

We arrived back in County Tyrone, Strabane, at the height of The Troubles in Northern Ireland in 1969. I was 8 years old. Strabane is a Catholic border town. I became aware of the contrast between the poorer Catholic back streets compared to the more opulent Protestant houses and farms in the area. I quickly adapted to my old community again and identified with Catholics as I tended to naturally identify with the oppressed, but didn't quite understand why at that time.

After my 11 plus examination however, the school with the better reputation was a Protestant one and so I left the familiar context of my Catholic primary school for the Protestant grammar school. From then on, I was taught from the opposite perspective of the sectarian divide and was part of the other community. I remember children from the Catholic estate pelting us with bricks and stones during our weekly cross-country class run. This was a complete turn about from my primary school days, when my friends and I used to throw stones and bricks that we got from the wall separating playground and cemetery at the army vehicles passing by the school playground. Being confused and a little frightened, I said nothing of my past. To people who had asked me my religion I replied, 'I'm Sikh.' Those daring enough went on and asked: 'Is that a Catholic Sikh or a Protestant Sikh?'

Pitaji was a travelling draper. He was well liked by both communities who had mythologized him as one of the first migrants in 1949. Often alone to look after six children on and off when Bibbiji had to go back to Punjab, over the years, he became also a violent alcoholic, who among other things shouted abuse and threatened us in Panjabi. Swearing in Panjabi was always more powerful than English. So I associated Panjabi with threat, violence, shame and fear from my dad as well as with Sikh pride, battling spirit, bravery and fighting for justice and equality, rooted in Sikh history and stories, which Pitaji told us as children.

But Panjabi was also my family language, the language of Punjab of India, the language of the group, of the extended family. Panjabi for me paradoxically became suffused with nurture, gentleness, security, which Bibbiji and my sisters represented, spiritual music in the Sikh readings and hymns that Pitaji sang and played on the harmonium on Sundays.

When I closed the front door, I was in a world of Panjabi. However, when I was alone with my sister or my brother in the home, we spoke English to each other. Not only was there a separation between the inside and outside, there was also a separation between the younger and older members of the family. I remember feelings of embarrassment as Pitaji talked to us in Panjabi in front of Irish people. People used to laugh at us – not out of spite, but out of mild shock. We were among the few Asians in Ireland at that time and as a family, we were treated like strange, exotic people.

However, my dad decided for the second time to send me and one of my sisters back to India in 1973 because he wanted us to be more Indian as is natural. Naturally also, I did not want to go. As children, we liked our life in Ireland, as it was the only life we knew. I had friends and enjoyed the community I lived in, even though it was split and violent. In Strabane when at school, I was a different character. I became one of the lads. I had friends and I felt they were badly needed. I came out of my shell. So Panjabi became identified with being closed in. I was kind of a rebel but passive when teachers were around, I was loud and gesticulated wildly in their absence. I was a clown. I felt more energetic and outgoing. I spoke much more. I loved the 'craic' (humorous conversation).

I was 12 years old when I went back to India, supposedly for good, once again. I was devastated. In fact, it was a stay for nine months. I was having trouble coping with the school at the foothills of the Himalayas and argued with my mother. I convinced her to let me go back to Strabane to live with my father, until I turned 14.

Without his wife, however, Pitaji had become increasingly frustrated, angry and more violent at being isolated and in fact became mentally disturbed. He made the decision to go back to India. He entrusted my care, and that of my sister (who had returned unmarried from India), to one of his four elder daughters. She had been educated and married an Irishman she met at university. She lived in Nottingham.

Entering my sister's household in Nottingham was a world apart from my Irish-Panjabi world. I became socialized into a mixed-race, multicultural, university-educated household, a world apart from white working class council house estate Panjabi/Irish upbringing. I came from a world full of the whirlwind of noise, from an action-packed drama where the daytime resonated with screams and shouts of the adults under stress and the night time was owned by the horrific flik-flak of army helicopter blades above the rooftops. In Nottingham, bookish silence reigned.

A provincial boy from a small Irish town, I grew increasingly self-conscious, as I contrasted my sister and her husband's impeccable English with my simple language. In Nottingham, I went to a large comprehensive school. It was so different from the schools I went to in Strabane because it was much bigger. I came into contact with a different type of racism, of a much more threatening kind. The kids at the school couldn't understand my broad Strabane accent, nor could the teachers. I got called a 'Paki-Paddy' and this label stuck. Within a month I had the perfect Nottingham accent. I can't remember having any difficulties with language during those years. I switched easily between all three identities.

The problem arose when the separate worlds met. I spoke my 'true' voice, the accent of Strabane, when at home at my sister's house, and I spoke another vernacular outside at school. When my friends came home, both worlds collided under the watchful eyes of my sister and her husband, or so I imagined. I felt an impostor, living a double life/identity once more, pretending to be English outside of the home, Irish inside of home and Panjabi somewhere else. My new male role model, my sister's husband, was and is a man of great integrity, loyalty and material generosity, whom I have always looked up to. He was also prone to anger and frustration. Although in hindsight, this anger was not directed at me, I somehow took it on as one more proof of my inadequacy. I construed this as a fatherly rejection, as Pitaji's last words to me, at Heathrow Airport had been 'I am not your father: Tom, my son-in-law, is now your father'. Tom's verbal outbursts reminded me of Pitaji's violence and paralysed me. Yet again, I found myself wanting in his eyes, as I was wanting in the eyes of Pitaji. I was convinced he saw my chameleon-like adaptation and frozen smile as cowardice.

My relationship with my father had always been problematic. I grew up deeply aware of having let him down. I was extremely passive in the face of his alcoholic violence. I was frightened. I had never been a sturdy child, having had frequent attacks of asthma as a kid, in sharp contrast to my healthier elder brother. I was skinny and often in and out of hospitals. The tradition of Sikh male is to be strong and with a fighting spirit. My father – orphaned early on – was such a fighter and he must have been deeply disappointed with me. While my elder brother got praised for his physical strength and stature, I think that my physical weakness embarrassed him. I was hit by him perhaps even more than the rest of my siblings. As a result, I cannot remember having ever received any affirmation and encouragement of my maleness by my father. Therefore, part of my struggle with my identity is also partly a struggle over the gender. People appreciate my kindness, softness and sensitivity – these traits I share with my sisters and am deeply grateful for. They stand me in good stead I suppose in a world where males are often complained about because they can't 'communicate'. I think, I can do that and indeed people come to me to share their burdens. I empathize easily.

On the other hand, my male identity is much more problematic. Aphasia has forced me to question how I define being a male. Perhaps, as I am writing this, I realize that losing Panjabi to some extent and the Irish vernacular somehow has pushed me away from the Sikh and Irish concept of maleness, which were promoted to me by my father and my sister's husband.

Having aphasia, by looking inward instead of outward, has also simplified my life by forcing me to make a choice between multiple identities acted out through languages. Paradoxically this is an exhilarating experience, and yet also an experience which has a sense of loss, of being shut out of my extended Panjabi family. My maturity has been arrested. In fact, this has been a theme of my life. Raised mainly by what, in hindsight, were over-protective women, I have found it easier to let them make sense of my life and let them take the decisions for me. This has antagonized the males in my family who saw me as a mammy's boy.

Part of my struggle with my identity is also struggling to grow up. My Panjabi family and my sisters protect me but also keep me around for protection for various reasons. But the Panjabi side of the family do not involve me in any serious discussions – I am too slow – I am not one of the adults. I remain a child forever. I could have hoped as I matured to resolve the many internal conflicts I had by talking to members of my Panjabi family and getting to know them as adults. Instead I am finding it difficult. It is not so much the younger generation. I can speak to them in English. It is the older generation, which represents my origins and my ancestry. I, like an adolescent, think 'they don't understand my world'. It has always been problematic for me to grow up in the Panjabi world.

Now, with aphasia, it seems the choice is no longer mine. I have been refused an opportunity to grow up in my family. On other hand, I have been given a new opportunity to focus all my energies on growing up in my second language.

After my stroke and subsequent aphasia, I have developed an identity that is much more independent of my family. A year and a half after the stroke, my wife and I separated. Someone with disability from Sikh families from Panjab is well looked after in terms of security and nurture, but for me it's too claustrophobic, limiting choice and challenge. So I chose to be independent and moved to inner city Bradford, where it would be easier to access services I needed.

However I am still struggling to find a voice within those two distinct parts of my family. I feel that as a child, I was 'spoken for' often, whether in Panjabi or in English. My role has always been to listen and perhaps nurture members of my family. Aphasia has locked me into this role. I do not have much of a voice now in the Panjabi family community. I am protected by them, but silent. One example is the family tension over my possible claim to a share of land in Panjab. Yet again, nobody in the Panjabi community included me in the discussions that went on about the land. I find it too difficult to organize my thoughts. I couldn't contribute effectively to the discussion. My sister from Nottingham – my *loco parentis* – on picking up on the differing and conflicting standpoints and likely difficulties, took my side about the land issue and represented me to the family. She debriefed me about the problem but also asked me to trust her to handle it and say more or less nothing. So my Panjabi voice is gone and my English voice, as I have pointed out, is somebody else's voice. My work identity is developing slowly after my stroke and aphasia. This is the area of my life where the loss is probably the greatest. It won't be a surprise to the reader that I have always been interested in different cultures, different ways of looking at things. I have always had an affinity with children and studied to become a primary teacher. I then chose to specialize in multicultural education via a postgraduate degree course at Bradford College. Bradford's main ethnic minority is a Muslim community from Kashmir in which people speak a version of Panjabi-Urdu.

Part of my work, I decided, was to become a bridge between the world of school and home. I became an advisory teacher for multicultural education. I started to organize parents' meetings and teachers' evenings, which attracted funding. As a Panjabi speaker, I could reach into the homes of the Pakistani community by talking to women in particular, who spoke insufficient English to be actively involved in school. Their main fear was that their children would lose their connection to home and the language of their origin. My job, I felt, was to convince them that the world of education and the world of home were interlinked. The parents had no stake in the schools and felt the responsibility lay with schools. One aim with my job as I saw it, was to emphasize the links between Panjabi and English.

I think I did have some success. The families started to trust the school system more, as they saw me as an Indian subcontinent bilingual representative of their community working in this other world. My work with cultural differences had naturally led me to becoming involved in anti-racism as I saw this as the underlying issue. I became an activist, fighting for gender and race equality alike.

This work was instrumental in getting me to a position of deputy headteacher of a school with virtually no native English-speaking children, consisting mainly of pupils from the Pakistani community and a smaller number from other minority groups – Ukrainian, Polish and Latvian. In this post, a few months before my brain haemorrhage, I had initiated and organized what was hoped to become a fairly major oral history project which involved pupils from two schools doing interviews in the community and publishing their work in a range of media.

After my stroke, I decided to look for a job and asked the Work-Able Unit, run by the local council. The role of this agency is to train and find work for disabled people in Bradford, to find them a position. They came up with a position as assistant teacher in an all-white school in a run-down estate in the city. In a way it suited me. I didn't feel I was in a position to advise anyone any more on anything much. I didn't have the language skills. This was only two years after my brain haemorrhage and a few months on from the third operation. My English was still coming back to me. But what it also meant is that I found myself in a situation I had not experienced since being a child and teenager in Ireland and Nottingham, where I went to an all-white school. My work as multicultural teacher, which enabled me to reclaim my Panjabi identity and link it to my English identity, was irrevocably lost.

Nonetheless, I am happier with my identity than I have been for a long time. I have a new partner, who is French and very individualist in the way she approaches life, perhaps not a coincidence, given my history. I am learning many things through my aphasia and appreciate the insights it gives me. For example, with aphasia I get a sense of an idea and it remains opaque, like seeing through a frosted glass, without precise definition. Or a concept wrapped in cellophane seen from afar. There is much effort involved in finding a word, and often I will forget why I was looking for it in the first place. I then use logic to retrace the steps that led me to the word. But it's something more than that. It's like a cross between going over the same ground, sometimes quite laterally (as I guess some people do) and a word that has the same rhythm or rhyme to it. Of course it helps if I relax. I also began to see the value of momentary silence when two people are relating through talking. You need language to define things, to fix things. But the obverse is also true. One cannot take another meaning because the meaning is fixed.

The use of language both gives rise to and kills meaning. Words label. Words can name and create meaning, bringing experience and understanding. However, they capture precisely what 'is', and not as an adage as experienced by that individual at that particular time. They are abstract maps and not sensory reality – moving instantly to objectify without allowing the subjective (in other words, the emotional truth experienced by that individual) to settle. Whereas aphasia allows me time to just 'be'.

Since 1999, I have been training to become a psychotherapist. As such, I am encouraged to be sensitized to go beyond 'empathy' (which involves verbal communication) and pick up emotions, which are pre-verbal, and this 'attunement' occurs at the earlier, infant atavistic level.

I wonder whether aphasia gives me an advantage here. I have discovered that my energies are directed more towards the emotional than the cognitive, thereby lessening control over what is eventually uttered. In addition, as I find it difficult to speak when emotionally charged, I assume that, in my interactions with people and my clients, I am allowing even more time for speech to form and become grounded.

As I write this, I am reading Greenberg's (1997) account of Freud and his aphasia book. Freud's early work on aphasia and neurology was influenced by Hughings Jackson, in particular in his theory of 'dissolution'. Jackson's theory on language, which we take for granted now, briefly states that the last-acquired are more advanced, thus the least organized capacities are lost before the earliest-acquired, the more habitual ones. And I would add these early experiences with language are saturated with emotion. We need to look within and pay close attention to our experience. We can perhaps hesitate to name our experience. Perhaps we do it too quickly, thereby imposing meaning on it and losing a chance to learn from it. I'm no linguist but I think aphasia in both languages helps me here.

Thinking back on what Bibbiji said when she first saw me after my stroke and proclaimed that I was atoning for the sins of past incarnations, I wonder what my family karma is? Perhaps it is about this notion of life as struggle, as punishment. In our family, we are never allowed to relax for a moment, in the knowledge that the next calamity is around the corner. Somehow, I have never seen my aphasia as a punishment. Lately, as I explained, I have seen it as an opportunity to create a new identity for myself, to question the meaning of words. The struggle with my identity is framed now.

I have always been a keen runner throughout my life, running away from stress, often it seemed, towards exhaustion, forgetfulness and finally peace. Aphasia simplified my life, like a run. Aphasia helped me break the family karma. Punishments are not always followed by another punishment – aphasia may be a curse for Bibbiji, is not a curse for me.

References

Greenberg, V. (1997) *Freud and His Aphasia Book: Language and the Sources of Psychoanalysis*. Cornell: Cornell University Press.

3

Talking to ourselves: dialogues in and out of language

Maria Black and Chris Ireland

Key points

- Chris is a teacher, counsellor and a poet. She has aphasia.
- Maria is a teacher and a linguist. She speaks different languages.
- In this chapter they talk together about their experiences of language and how language affects thinking.
- Chris and Maria think inner language (the way we talk to ourselves) is important as well as external language (what we say out loud).
- Inner language helps us to pay attention to thoughts and do things with thoughts, like remembering, comparing, linking two different thoughts.
- Inner language can be affected both by aphasia and when a person moves between two different languages.
- Sometimes Maria feels in limbo – between two languages. Sometimes Chris feels like she is in a foreign language that she can't quite grasp.
- They talk about some of the things that make it hard or helpful to pin down and get a clear shape for thoughts and emotions and meanings.
- For example, sometimes in quick conversations other people don't listen carefully and they miss the point; Chris sometimes finds seeing words or saying words aloud helps her to check it out.
- Chris and Maria play with different words and say that connections between words and sounds and meanings can be creative and poetic.
- They think there should be more attention to helping people with aphasia explore their inner language in therapy and research.

Who are we
. . .
who must read our own history
in another tongue,
follow the butterfly
of our being
across maps of imagination
trying to recreate
the lost structure
of our soul?

        (Jimmy Story 1998)

Introduction

In spite of the extensive literature on aphasia, talking to oneself, one of the most frequent and common uses of language, is rarely discussed. It is still true, as Vygotsky pointed out, that 'the whole inward aspect of language, the side turned towards the person, not towards the outer world, has been so far an almost unknown territory' (Vygotsky 1962: 152).

'Inner speech' has many uses that can vary depending on the activity, the situation and the person. Nevertheless, all of us use internal language to mediate and make conscious some of our thinking (Sokolov 1972; Kinsbourne 2000). So why is there so little discussion of the effects of aphasia on inner language and inner life?

There are several reasons for this neglect. First, there are the methodological difficulties of investigating inner language and thinking. Second, people with aphasia have been given few opportunities to introspect and share their experiences (see Parr *et al.* 1997; Ireland and Black 1992). Third, certain assumptions about aphasia have got in the way of more detailed investigations of the relationship between aphasia, inner language and thinking.

Aphasia is primarily seen as a problem of linguistic communication with other people. 'External' language is what assessment and therapy tend to concentrate on. This strategy is understandable as the impact of a communication disability is enormous. Nevertheless, we should not neglect the consequences of aphasia for inner language and thinking.

In this chapter, we try to map out the 'almost unknown territory' of inner language. The chapter is a dialogue between two people who have a theoretical, professional interest in language as well as direct experience of moving in and out of language – through aphasia for Chris Ireland, and multilingualism for Maria Black.

Our experiential exploration leads us to several conclusions:

- Language, internal or external, is *not the same* as thought. Thinking can take place when language is disrupted, not fully acquired or rarely used.
- Aphasia and shifting between languages, however, *can affect inner language and our ability to talk to ourselves.*
- Although not the same as thought, inner language allows us to *pay attention to our thoughts, to keep hold of them, compare and link them together* to form more complex thoughts, arguments and plans.
- Not all aspects of thinking are equally affected by disruptions of language: *some thoughts are easier* to reconstruct and hold than others.
- *Talking to ourselves*, in whatever form we do it, *is important not only cognitively but emotionally.* It can be a source of pleasure and creativity.
- Facilitating a *person's internal dialogue should be part of therapy and social support.*

We signpost our exploration by reference to some of the theories, old and new, that have helped us understand, keep hold of and articulate our experiences. These theories, we believe, provide a useful basis for further exploration and experimentation.

We chose a dialogue format for several reasons. First, it most closely reflected the way we work together: it is an interaction of equals with different experiences and contributions. Both of us provide 'data' for discussion and analyse these data with methods and theories we are familiar with. In the interaction, further insights and questions emerge – a dialogue allowed us to represent this dynamic more directly and explicitly.

As the theme of our exploration was the relationship between thinking and language, it seemed particularly important to show that someone with aphasia is not just a 'source of data' or a vivid witness to the experience but an equal contributor to the analysis itself. In this sense too, we wanted to link back to the tradition of Soviet neuropsychologists like Luria, who took seriously the insights of people with aphasia and integrated them with other methods of investigation.

The dialogue format also allowed us to maintain our individual styles of speaking and use informal language, while occasionally bringing in some technical terms and theoretical references. We wanted to find a common ground where personal experience and theoretical analysis could fit together, making our exploration more accessible and relevant to a wider range of readers, with and without aphasia.

The dialogue in this piece is woven out of the threads of many taped or transcribed conversations. We selected the observations and examples that seemed most reliable and consistent in that they regularly surfaced in a similar form over many occasions. Most of our exploration is based on introspection, which, as William James said, is 'difficult and fallible', though not necessarily more so than other methods of observation. In dealing with issues like 'internal language', some introspecting is inescapable, as it is in many other areas of theory and practice. For instance, we could not provide adequate sight correction without introspective judgements by the people whose eyesight is measured. Without introspection how would one answer 'Do you see better with this lens or with that?' Like Chafe (1994: 14), we would argue that 'A more balanced approach would recognize, not just the difficulty, but also the validity of private observations, joining the ghost of William James in seeing what can be done about incorporating them into systematic research' (see also Kinsbourne 2000).

This chapter is just a first step towards more systematic research.

The dialogue

MB: Most of what I read about the relationship between language and thinking left me unsatisfied. It did not convince me theoretically and, perhaps more importantly here, it did not describe my experience of moving from one language I knew well to another I was learning. I wanted to understand the linguistic limbo of that transition – something akin to the experience of aphasia. It was probably the most useful training in aphasia I had. But the similarities and links between the two types of experience were rarely discussed in the aphasia literature.

I came to London on my own when I was 19, in 1970. I had already much experience of the pleasures and problems of moving between two languages as I grew up in a household and city where both Italian and Piedmontese were spoken. Piedmontese is quite different from Italian, closer to the languages of southern France or northern Spain. I did not speak Piedmontese myself but it was spoken to me all the time and I understood it. Both languages were part of me in a way I did not really understand then.

When I arrived here, I had enough English to operate on a practical level and communicate quite effectively. I was a product of the enormous socio-economic changes taking place in Italy in the 1950s and 1960s: the daughter of rural migrants from a peasant background and with very little education, I had been well educated. I was a voracious reader with a long-standing interest in writing and language. I was keen to learn English quickly and make it my own, to leave not only Italy but Italian behind.

There was a period, or maybe several periods or phases, when I was operating in a language where, as you said, 'my thoughts and emotions are so much bigger and quicker than my language tools' (Ireland and Black 1992). There was no question for me that thinking and language were distinct: there was so much going on in my head all the time and yet it could not find either its proper internal or external expression.

I don't know if people were aware of the mismatch between my thoughts and what I said. They reacted in the ways you and other people with aphasia often complain about: they would correct some aspect of pronunciation or grammar even when it did not make any difference to the meaning. As you said, 'If people knew what I am trying to say well enough to correct, why bother?' (Ireland and Black 1992).

On the other hand, they would rarely offer alternatives that could have improved the fit between my thoughts and their external expression. They would finish my sentences if I groped for the right words, usually assuming that the thoughts I was trying to convey were simpler and more basic than what I had in mind. What I realized then, which has been confirmed by many years of teaching linguistics, was that prejudice and preconceptions were not the only problem. The problem was also that *their* listening skills and conscious understanding of language needed developing – not just mine. Some of their reactions were more often due to not knowing what else to do than to negative attitudes.

CI: Yes, sometimes I foreign in my own language. People don't have time for deep listening. You grab conversations with people. On the hop conversations, I hate them. They hurt me. Stressed out my brain, too much in. Your head goes everywhere. People sometimes say words but they are not in touch with the emotional, the deep thoughts. On the hop, there is so much moulted stuff . . . multi . . . multi-layered stuff. Not enough time to check what they really mean by it. When I talk with you or Carole we have space. I get very excited and exhausted but it feels more containing. Rooted feeling, with space and quietness. Got time to unpacking it out. Sift through thoughts softly. I seek people to hold information for me, not like advocate but to hold me in a conversation. I can't hold so well now. Not only the information but the implication of what is being said – what's their bit and what's my bit.

MB: People often treat the link between thought and language as a static thing: it's either there or it's not. We should treat it as a dynamic process, as Vygotsky said, 'a continual movement back and forth from thought to word and from word to thought', an 'inner movement through a series of planes' (1962: 125). You'll like this: he said a thought could be 'compared to a cloud shedding a shower of words' (1962: 150).

CI: Wonderful, I want it for a poem!

MB: My linguistic transitions between Italian and English, and later English and Spanish, brought out another issue about the relationship between thinking and language that people with aphasia often mention. I was clear that thinking and language were not one and the same thing since my thoughts could be much more complex than my language. But I also had a sense that language wasn't just a mechanical translation of those thoughts to myself and to other people. To quote Vygotsky again, 'words cannot be put on by thought like a ready-made garment' (1962: 126). The unavailability or instability of my access to certain aspects of language made my thinking less available to me. I would find myself losing the sense of what the thought was, it would blur and slip through my mind's fingers as if it had not been quite there. Vygotsky really pinned that feeling down for me by saying that 'a thought unembodied in words remains a shadow'. I sometimes felt that my inner landscape was full of such shadows. I knew there was something there, that a process was going on but couldn't work out its precise shape and unfolding.

CI: Yes, I get that sometimes. There is a meaning in my head, I want it but I don't know what it is. So the only way I can handle that one is by writing it down to check it out. The only way is translating it through the pen. Then I think 'that looks fine' and sometimes 'that looks funny' but I don't know what the meaning was exactly or how to spell it. I might sound it out and then I know I had another word in my head, although I don't know what it is, how to say it, spell it or write it down. It's trapped there. I can get thoughts in my head that only makes sense if I write it down. I don't contain in my head. When I write down, I let it allow. Time, ripple, enjoy that phrase, soothe me, soft.

MB: So in those cases, it is really the thought and the particular meaning that are difficult to pin down, not just the form of words – their sounds or spellings.

CI: Is variable, doesn't always happen. Sometimes I hear myself. I'm much more aware of the language going on in my head, much more than before the stroke, partly because of the speech therapy, psychoanalysis and working with you. But when I'm thinking, concentrating, I hear more in my head. Somehow I enjoy the sound and also I try to search the words more appropriate the meaning. Sometimes I see what I hear in my mind, even though I don't know how to write it down. Sometimes I have to make it loud, I have to say it over vocally: 'Oh, that word?' It could be a little word or a mixed up word. When I'm able to know what that word is, particularly a mixed up one, I put it down on paper and allow myself being the silly word it is. Even it might be silly, it isn't 'cause it's quite complex. It's fertile ground.

MB: The cloud of thought has burst its shower of words to soften and prepare the ground?

CI: Yeah, I always allow the word to come out as much as I can. It might be a nonsense sound or letters but later it's not that much nonsense. I look at it and see what it could be: a bit of this and a bit of that, it's quite appropriate what it is.

MB: So there are always connections of thoughts, meanings, sounds and bits of orthography but until you have said aloud some of the sounds or have the letters in front of you, you don't know what all the connections are.

CI: Yes, I can only suss it out later. Yesterday I was trying to write a poem. It's called 'Words to *toast*', no, 'Words to *taste* in my London garden'. When I was in my garden, I been thinking how I like golden rod, lemon balm, mock orange, all taste. But what that called on fence? I kept going to it, still can't find the word on the fence! After a cup of tea, jasmine it was, oh yes, it was *honeysuckle* on the fence. I love words to taste.

MB: And your appreciation of words is expressed by both toasting and tasting them! You corrected yourself, as if you had made a phonological slip, but in fact the sound and visual similarities also bring forth a meaning connection – both *toast and taste* express appreciation and celebration. That's what makes your language so amazing and powerful: there are so many connections!

CI: That's what I sometime aware of and then I think 'oh, that's it, I keep that'. Sometimes I more clever than I think I was!

MB: But you always recognize the connections very quickly, even when you look surprised at discovering them. Your facial expression and intonation often suggest that you knew exactly what you were playing with. Yet you can only recognize your thoughts once you are saying them aloud or looking at the written words. It is as if you knew all the thought, meaning and form connections, and yet didn't know them.

CI: I like that idea, knowing and not knowing. It makes sense.

MB: Perhaps, in these cases, you know that thinking is going on but you don't know what you are thinking. Only the external language can bring the thoughts fully out of the shadows. The external forms have become necessary for communicating with yourself.

Your experience is similar to that of the people with aphasia described by Soviet neuropsychologists who claimed that internal language was also affected by aphasia. Luria and Sokolov, for instance, say that people with aphasia often 'perform various thought operations considerably better aloud than to themselves'

(Sokolov 1972: 63). Luria quotes a young man with aphasia who had greater difficulty with complex sentences and thinking when actual articulation was blocked:

I read it and it is as if I understand it, but cannot figure it out . . . But if I repeat it aloud, I understand. Then I can figure it out right away.

(Luria 1963, cited in Sokolov 1972: 63)

But it is very hard to stay with that knowing and not knowing, let alone make sense of it to anyone else. I also had that experience every time I moved from my main language to another. At first, when I'm thinking, I literally talk to myself aloud in the new language. Then I shift to a more internal 'sounding out'. The process quietens down but words still have a definiteness of shape they do not have when I'm thinking in my usual language. This happens not only when I shift from a language I know to one I'm learning but also when I go from my usual language to one I have not practised for a while. For me, it is exactly as Sokolov says:

As learning takes root and mental operations become increasingly automa- tized, the need for external verbalization (enunciation aloud) arises no longer, and it is replaced by reduced, abbreviated verbalization – inner speech.

(Sokolov 1972: 263)

So language, external or internal depending on the circumstances, can make our thinking available to us. It is not *the same* as thought nor is it *the only form* of thinking but it allows us to pay attention to our thinking. The cognitive linguist, Ray Jackendoff, talks about language giving us 'potential handles' by which attention 'grasps' and 'holds onto' concepts (Jackendoff 1997).

CI: There is also something about controlling the thinking, especially for me as a poet. When I can think 'So, that's to do with that meaning and that sound is to do with that other meaning', it's almost like the poet's voice coming stronger than would not have been without showing the 'errors' or whatever we call them. Write them down, they are tools. Play my mind. You have the friends of language, you feel good. That is a dialogue in itself. When it becomes conscious, it gives me power.

MB: Jackendoff would say that it gives you more processing power too. He argues that, by allowing us to pay attention to our thoughts, language anchors and stabilizes thought in short-term memory and makes it possible for us to process it in greater detail. We can then draw finer comparisons and make more complex connections between thoughts.

In one of our conversations, you captured the interaction

between thinking and language perfectly. 'Language roots my thinking', you said. When I asked you whether you meant *roots* or *routes*, you decided it was both. Like you, I need them both to make sense of my experience. Language seems to anchor my thinking and allow me to retrace my mental steps more directly.

Thinking feels quite different whenever I'm in between languages. The best way I can explain the difference is by analogy. When I was a child I used to see shapes in the wood of an old wardrobe. I saw the grain of one of its doors as a face – a scary face, a devil. If I felt anxious, I would arrive at the crucial spot cautiously and gradually, moving my eyes from place to place and reconstructing the shape as a purely visual process. I had to retrace my steps and find my route to the face-like shape again and again – there was no shortcut. When I felt more daring, I would whisper the word 'devil' to myself and straight away the word would conjure up the face out of the wood. Both methods got me to the same spot but the word was a more direct route and it never failed to get me there. Reconstructing my visual path was a more laborious, tortuous process and sometimes I got snared in irrelevant details, unable to find my way to the face. Whenever I've been in between languages, thinking felt like reconstructing a process from scratch over and over again, with little to root and route me.

CI: Yeah, when I really concentrate a word, it's fertile, lots of conducting, connecting images. But language can lurk in the back of the head and be nasty. Sometimes thoughts of language can become very powerful, like bullies. There is only one word and I really want to get it. How can I get that word? Awful, it hurts! Example: took two days after we talked about massage session. Relaxation, energy but lose it travelling back and other things. Think: *scar . . . scuff . . . squaid . . . squandling* ? Think on sound in head, sound out, write down, playing sounds and shapes. Use meaning 'waste', check dictionary. I want it to fit deeper for me. But I cannot find it, not a good one.

MB: In this case, it was the word itself that you were trying to track down. You nearly had it – I'm assuming you wanted the verb *squander.* When that happens, though, one can get so lost en route to the word that the thought itself blurs and disappears.

When we are thinking about more concrete things, it is often easier to fall back on connected sensory or perceptual codes – look how you recovered your train of thought and got the word 'honeysuckle' after a cup of jasmine tea. The psychologist William James talks about trying to remember a name. 'The state of our consciousness is peculiar,' he says. 'There is a gap therein, but no mere gap. It is a gap that is intensely active' (1950: 251).

If we are thinking about more abstract relations, such as complex actions or states, there is still 'a gap' in our consciousness but it feels to me like a different sort of gap. When we can't get the words that code those relations, it becomes extremely difficult to hold on to the thinking and truly know what we think. That is why the transition between languages often feels like a cognitive, as well as linguistic, limbo. Maybe we should add another verb to your definition of how thinking and language interact: language can root, route *and* rout *thinking!* That the crucial words in your definition are all verbs, or so-called 'predicates', is appropriate since it is usually verbs that code more abstract relations (see Black and Chiat 2000, and 2003).

Luria and Sokolov were probably the first to connect 'the extreme paucity of verb forms' with disruptions of inner language and thinking in particular forms of aphasia (see Sokolov 1972; Luria 1973). I've only just rediscovered their recommendation that 'special attention must therefore be given to the restoration of the predicative aspect of inner speech' (Sokolov 1972: 64).

They were well ahead of their times in trying to find methods to support inner language and thinking as part of speech and language therapy. This is something implicit in many current therapies but rarely made explicit or discussed. We also need some therapy for inner language or 'thinking therapy' (Black 2002).

I don't think I could have coped with the loneliness of my first few months in London without all that talking and writing to myself. You have often stressed the importance of being supported in reconstructing your thinking through an examination of sounds, letters, bits of words and connections between words. As you, and many writers and poets have pointed out, inner dialogue is a form of poetry, of creativity. I think Yeats said something like, 'Rhetoric is the argument you have with another, poetry, with oneself.'

CI: What I found now is I can do something better than before. I'm enjoying words, rhythms. Poetry is the only thing that soothes me, other than massage. Is something feed, massage my soul and my mind as well. The poetry is the most containing of all the things I've done. Feels like washing my mindthoughts with an inner rhythm: ripple, ripple, still, still. Balming sounds, worm waves in head. Catch web-dream words on touch, torch paper. Oh, got a poem starting!

Conclusion

We have argued that aphasia, like moving between languages, can affect our 'internal language'. This, in turn, can impact on our ability to pay attention to our thoughts, hold on to them and combine them. Thinking, planning and talking to ourselves can become more awkward and slippery. If we are correct, aphasia therapy, social support and self-help should include strategies to deal with problems of internal as well as external language.

Internal processes, as opposed to overt behaviour, have already regained theoretical respectability thanks to modern neuropsychology and psycholinguistics. As Kinsbourne (2000: 120) points out, the last century 'has witnessed an inward gradient of research focus, from overt behaviour, through the internal models of the cognitive revolution, to a *fin de siecle finale* of swelling interest in consciousness'. A shift of focus to internal language and thinking could be the next step, as Kinsbourne predicts. Related changes could occur in therapy and social support. This, however, would require a major shift in attitude: communication with oneself would have to be treated as seriously as communication with others.

References

Black, M. (2002) Therapy for thinking and rethinking therapy, in L. Battistin, M. Dam and P. Tonin (eds) *Proceedings of the 3rd World Congress on Neurological Rehabilitation*, 2–6 April, Venice, Italy.

Black, M. and Chiat, S. (2000) Putting thoughts into verbs: developmental and acquired impairments, in W. Best, K. Bryan, and J. Maxim (eds) *Semantic Processing: Theory and Practice*. London: Whurr Publishers.

Black, M. and Chiat, S. (2003) Noun–verb dissociations: a multi-faceted phenomenon, *Journal of Neurolinguistics*, 16, 231–250.

Chafe, W. (1994) *Discourse, Consciousness and Time*. Chicago: University of Chicago Press.

Ireland, C. and Black, M. (1992) Living with aphasia: the insight story, *UCL Working Papers in Linguistics*, 4: 355–8.

Jackendoff, R. (1997) *The Architecture of the Language Faculty*. Cambridge, MA: MIT Press.

James, W. (1950) *Principles of Psychology*. New York: Rinehart, Holt and Winston.

Kinsbourne, M. (2000) Inner speech and the inner life, *Brain and Language*, 71: 120–3.

Luria, A.R. (1973) *The Working Brain*. Harmondworth: Penguin Books.

Parr, S., Byng, S. and Gilpin, S. (1997) *Talking about Aphasia*. Buckingham: Open University Press.

Sokolov, A.N. (1972) *Inner Speech and Thought*. New York: Plenum Press.

Story, Jimmy (1998) New rom, in I. Hancock, S. Dow and R. Djuric (eds) *The Roads of the Roma: The PEN Anthology of Gipsy Writers*. Hatfield: University of Hertfordshire Press.

Vygotsky, L.S. (1962) *Thought and Language*. Cambridge, MA: MIT Press.

4

A time of transition: a matter of control and confidence

Sue Boazman

Key points

- Sue Boazman is a counsellor and a person with aphasia.
- In this chapter she talks about her personal experience of stroke, aphasia and epilepsy.
- She says her recovery did not go up in a straight line but went up and down.
- Sue thinks the ups and downs were closely related to feelings of control and confidence. For example, when she suddenly had an epileptic fit she lost all sense of control; a bad experience on a course made a big dent in her confidence and that made her speech worse too.
- After her stroke Sue trained to be a counsellor and she now works with people who have had strokes.
- Sue thinks some counsellors and therapists need to pay more attention to the everyday ups and downs in the lives of those with aphasia.
- She recommends that counsellors think about their clients' confidence and feelings of control.

As a counsellor I am often aware that the general thinking around the concept of recovery is that it goes in a straight line. In my personal experience as someone with aphasia this is not so. My progress has been varied, sometimes up and sometimes down, with no particular pattern. In my case, these variations depended very much on the levels of control and confidence I was experiencing.

In this chapter, I will explore the many changes that have taken place for me since I had my stroke 13 years ago. These transitions have sometimes been complex and painful, and sometimes enlightening and wonderful! What I am describing here is my own experience. It is not intended to be a model for others to be guided by, but more a description of my personal journey. My own philosophy is that each person is a unique individual and so what you read in the following pages may work for me, but not for you.

My stroke affected my speech and language, my physical abilities, and later resulted in epilepsy. Having aphasia and a physical disability is something I have learned to live with over the years. Yet, somehow, it no longer feels like a label – more a state of being.

In this chapter, I will explore how this new state of being has become my reality. This includes the challenge of developing epilepsy and my personal development through training to be a counsellor. Becoming epileptic as a result of my stroke was very damaging to my confidence and self-esteem and felt like an even greater hurdle to overcome than the actual stroke itself. In the beginning, I had absolutely no control over my seizures and this generated all sorts of fears and fantasies for me.

My development as counsellor has played an enormous part in my personal growth and development. Through many, many hours of self-reflection, I have become more familiar with the way that I work and what makes me do the things that I do.

To me, the amount of control and confidence that I have experienced at different times has played a vital part in my transition. In this chapter I will consider the balance between control and confidence and how these can be influenced by external factors, which are not necessarily caused by physical disability and aphasia.

Beginnings

Before my stroke I had been employed by a computer company. During the ten years that I worked with the firm, I had progressed from being an administrator to becoming a supervisor and then a manager. My self-esteem and self-confidence had grown through the years, and I knew that my colleagues valued my opinions and suggestions. At home my husband, Bill, and I had role-swapped six months before and so he was looking after our two children, Kelly aged 4, and Lucie who was 2. Life was good. I was at a stage where I felt fully competent and fully in control of my life. Then, in a split second my whole life changed for good.

As I was driving home from work one evening, I felt a strange fizzing noise in my head. It got worse, and I was forced to pull over into a lay-by until it subsided. Suddenly, my right side collapsed and I was left hanging onto the steering wheel with my left hand. My thoughts at this stage were very composed. I experienced no sense of panic because my main objective at this stage was to get out of the car somehow. Looking back I managed this situation in the way I had been trained to in my job – I took control. I remained conscious until I was safely in an ambulance and then I lapsed into unconsciousness for the next two weeks.

I woke up with my head swathed in bandages, recovering from a seven hour operation to clip the aneurysm in my brain. As I became more aware of my new circumstances in hospital, I began to realize that all control had been relinquished to the nursing staff and consultants in charge of my case. The busy life I had been used to, where I had been so competent and able, did not exist any more. I quickly became resentful, angry and frustrated. This was compounded by the fact that I had become paralysed down my right side and could no longer speak.

I quickly realized that to regain my speech was all-important. My physical progress was slow, but somehow to conquer aphasia became my priority. As I saw it, my speech was like a reflection of my personality, the very core of my being and vital to my sanity. Yet, strangely enough, I was completely unaware of the gravity of my situation. The nursing sister told me that I would always be in a wheelchair, never speak again and that the only way I would be able to communicate would be by writing with my left hand. This news was given to me about four weeks after my stroke and it simply did not register with me. I was convinced that I would be in good health and fully fit within six months.

I sometimes became conscious of putting on a brave face for the benefit of my husband and children and the rest of my family. My background as a manager had taught me to 'manage' my situation and I looked on this dilemma as merely a temporary setback. At this point maintaining a positive attitude worked for me. Denying my true feelings gave me the courage and confidence to carry on regardless. It did not matter to me that some therapists thought I was being unrealistic. What did matter was my own mindset, my total and unfailing belief that my situation was only temporary.

Recovery

I spent the next nine months in and out of rehabilitation where I was able to concentrate on my speech and language and regaining some physical ability. In fact, I spent only a few weeks in a wheelchair, quickly recovering my balance and mobility to the point where I no longer needed it. Through becoming more independent, I began to feel a sense of being in control again. I worked hard at my speech and language with my therapist who had the special ability to let me find my own limitations, without enforcing her own agenda. I later came to appreciate that this was an exceptional quality and one that created total trust between us. By the time I came out of rehabilitation I had begun to realize that both my communication and physical disability were likely to be permanent, in spite of continuing gradual improvement.

New challenges

After coming out of rehabilitation I was busy concentrating on practical issues like washing and ironing, cooking and housework and generally taking care of my family. But worse was still to come. About a year after my stroke, I contracted epilepsy as a result of the surgery I had had in hospital. This hit me very hard in all kinds of ways.

The first seizure was a *grand mal*. I had acquired another label. I was now 'epileptic'. This was harder for me to deal with than the actual stroke. With the stroke, I was making a good recovery and I could see and feel progress, physically and mentally. I was beginning to feel more confident and in control once more. With the epilepsy, I was suddenly thrust into the unknown – and worse still, the confidence that I had struggled so hard to regain had once more deserted me.

I didn't know when the next seizure would occur. They came with little or no warning and I became terrified to go out of the house in case I would have a seizure in the street. I saw my doctor who prescribed medication to control my seizures. Time and time again I would 'forget' to take my tablets. This would result in another seizure. Some people may label this as denial, that I was ignoring the problem and pretending that it didn't exist. However I would suggest a different interpretation. Before my stroke I did not have to rely on tablets and, at this stage, I was still desperately trying to regain some semblance of my old lifestyle. Because epilepsy was something I had no control over perhaps what I was actually doing was attempting to seize control of my life. I learnt the hard way that taking my medication on a regular basis meant that I would not have to endure the seizures. After several months I began to realize that taking my medication reliably meant that I could be in control once more.

About two years after my stroke my working life faded into the distance although at this stage I was still eager to remind others around me that before my stroke I had been a manager! On reflection the whole point of making this statement was to emphasize that a short while ago I had held a responsible and highly active job. The purpose of calling attention to my previous status was to strengthen my self-esteem and re-affirm my competence to myself.

Gradually I began to realize that although I was doing well on the practical side something was missing and I needed emotional support from a source other than my family. As time went on, accessing both this emotional support and some form of new personal challenge became my highest priority. As I became more aware of these needs I began to lapse into bouts of mild depression. I had been officially retired from work on a long-term disability basis and now I clearly needed a purpose in my life other than being a housewife. I needed something to tax my brain once more, a challenge that would stretch and invigorate me.

Turning points

In 1993 I took a short bereavement and loss counselling course that helped me to reflect on and understand the processes that I was going through. This was a revelation to me! The course used the professional language that I recognized and reminded me of the way I had been treated before my stroke. People were interested in me as a person and not on account of my disability. I felt that my opinions were respected and that I was valued as an individual once more. I clung on desperately. Returning to familiar ground allowed me to feel in control again and, with a greater sense of control, some of my former confidence started to return.

I began to realize that it was these two vital factors, control and confidence, that were making the difference. In the three years since my stroke, my life had been like a rollercoaster. I had battled constantly to keep my head above water. With so many new and totally different situations to get used to it was no wonder that control and confidence had taken a temporary back seat. For the first time since I was a child I had become dependent once more. I had to learn to speak again, walk again and cope with the stigma, both real and imagined, of becoming epileptic. Therefore when for the first time I developed a sense of renewed control and confidence I realized how important these feelings were to my general well-being. These two factors also played an invaluable role in raising my overall self-esteem.

This new understanding led me to seek counselling for myself. Although my counsellor had no personal experience of stroke, she seemed to have great empathy for my pain and emotional distress. My husband and family were very supportive, but they were too close and I needed someone who was more remote. The relief was immense! Here was somebody that I could talk to in private, who wouldn't judge me and who wouldn't offer advice. I didn't want these types of help. I just wanted someone to listen while I came to my own conclusions and decisions in my own time. I entered into a long-term contract with my counsellor which from time to time still continues today.

Counselling helped me to explore and understand the processes that were happening inside me and this was my particular turning point. I realized that feeling confused, frustrated, elated and then depressed again were all natural feelings for somebody who has survived any traumatic event. This realization in itself was an immense relief. It confirmed that I was not going mad and that all these emotions that I was encountering were, in fact, perfectly normal. With my growing self-esteem, my self-image began to change, and gradually I began to see myself as a worthwhile human being again.

In 1995 I embarked on a three-year psychodynamic counselling course that taught me a lot about aspects of my own core personality and behaviour patterns. During this period I became more confident, proving to myself that I was capable of learning and growing again. This felt good. Throughout the course, I saw a more reflective side of my personality developing and became more at ease with my aphasia and my physical disability. In 1997 I embarked on an Advanced Diploma in Integrative Counselling and during this course I began to increase my skills in other areas. I began developing the ability look outside myself no longer needing to concentrate solely on my own self-image and self-esteem.

Control and confidence – charting a course

The following charts show my own perception of how separate life events affected my aphasia and, as a consequence, my sense of control and confidence. In Figures 4.1 and 4.2, I attempt to represent visually how my aphasia, physical disability and epilepsy interacted over time with my feelings of control and confidence. The vertical line from 0 to 100 corresponds to the percentage of confidence and control I was feeling at that time. The horizontal line represents the years, broken down into six-month periods.

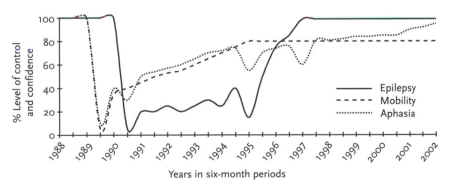

Figure 4.1 Levels of control and confidence linked with my aphasia, mobility and epilepsy

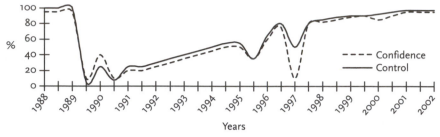

Figure 4.2   Levels of control and confidence 1988–2002

My aphasia relates very closely to my perceived levels of control and confidence with regard to various life events. I am convinced that my ability to express myself in a coherent way was directly affected by these feelings. It is noticeable (see Figure 4.1) that during the first year my level of control over my speech went roughly from about 0 to 50 per cent and with it, my sense of confidence about my ability to communicate. In 1991, when I had my first epileptic seizure, my confidence in my speech wavered slightly. It is interesting to note here how one disability (my epilepsy) impacted on another (my aphasia). As I experienced a loss of control and confidence with my epilepsy, so my control and confidence was lost with my aphasia. My own explanation is that epilepsy made me a focal point, drawing attention to my disabilities, while that was just what I was trying to avoid, particularly when I was also struggling to deal with my aphasia. It made me feel exposed and vulnerable.

During the next few years my ability to cope with aphasia improved. As this happened my confidence grew, and with it my sense of control. But then I experienced two significant setbacks. In 1995 my epilepsy became out of control again and as a consequence, I lost confidence in my speech. I had a series of major seizures accompanied by mild depression. During this period I felt a continual state of despair and I could not see a way forward. I finally realized that my epilepsy would be permanent and that was my turning point. I learnt that by taking my medication I could control my epilepsy and my life and so finally I began to take it on a regular basis. Consequently the seizures began to stabilize. At last I began to see the light at the end of the tunnel. For the last six years I have been totally free from any kind of seizure and my confidence and feeling of control has steadily risen.

However, in 1997 I experienced another setback. I had been on a three-year part-time psychodynamic counselling course and had completed both written and practical components of the course well. I was very surprised therefore when a major problem arose during the final assessment. The assessor made specific reference to my aphasia and difficulty with speech. In her written assessment she bluntly pointed out:

My doubts about her working as a psychodynamic counsellor, stem from one aspect of her physical disability which is her difficulty in finding words, particularly when she is under pressure, stress or anxiety. How a client will feel about Sue, who has a speech disability is an important issue.

The content of that assessment effectively prevented me from becoming a counsellor with that particular organization. This was a devastating blow to my confidence and sense of control, simultaneously (see Figure 4.2). When this happened my speech got noticeably worse (see Figure 4.1). I would forget what I was saying mid-sentence and my word-finding difficulties got markedly worse. Close friends and even acquaintances also noticed this deterioration in my speech. However, this time, I recovered quickly and I was able to view this setback as only temporary. Perhaps I was able to see it in this way because recent experience had taught me that I had successfully overcome other major traumas in my life, such as my stroke and epilepsy. I had visualized becoming a counsellor for so long that it was fast becoming my reality. I took stock of my situation and within six months successfully applied for and was accepted on an alternative counselling course.

As my training progressed, I started to notice a whole variety of trans-formations taking place which must have evolved from my growing sense of control and confidence. With a new skill set that I could incorporate into my daily life, I was beginning to feel more complete as a person. Now I saw myself as a more reflective individual with a clearer understanding of my needs and a continuing desire to grow and change. Independence, my own self-image and my self-esteem seemed to harmonize once more and I felt that I had completed the circle.

Moving forward

To conclude, I wish to put a controversial spanner in the works! Classic grief models suggest that there are four key stages or tasks in moving forward from grief and loss:

Task 1: accepting the reality of the loss
Task 2: experiencing the pain of grief
Task 3: adjusting to the loss
Task 4: moving on

These models tend to promote a particular and rather fixed way of thinking about loss. In my opinion the experience of loss associated with a sudden acquired disability does not always follow such a well trodden path. For many people, myself included, the sense of loss and bereave-ment linked with sudden acquired disability may take a very different course. It seems evident that when people face sudden disability life changes and circumstances may play a very strong role in moving forward, sometimes at odds with more typical trends in grieving. For example, some of my clients who come for counselling show no signs of anger linked to their sudden acquired disability. Yet, according to current models, one of the most common signs of loss and bereavement is anger. In my opinion it would be dangerous to assume that because these feelings are absent, the person is going through some sort of denial. Denial is an over-used term, perhaps reflecting more the simplistic perspective of the health and rehabilitation 'expert' than the experience of the person who is living through the complexities of change. Obviously there may be times when you *are* in true denial, but also times when 'denial' is a false and meaningless label, applied without thought for or exploration of multiple, complex feelings and reactions. In these cases 'denial' could be more to do with the limited imagination of an 'expert' than any real understanding of an individual's internal reality.

In my own case my growing and interacting level of control and confidence was paramount to my overall recovery. So, what do the terms control and confidence mean to me? There is a subtle difference between the two. It seems that while control is a kind of check and balance system, confidence has more to do with feelings. My own interpretation (with the help of a dictionary!) is this: being in control of my life is a measurement of my own trust or belief (confidence) in myself.

As a counsellor working with people who have confronted sudden disability I have become increasingly aware that for some clients their own perceived level of control and confidence is paramount to their ability to work with a way of life that has become their new reality. For example, one of my clients, who has severe aphasia is usually accompanied by his wife on the one and a half hour journey to meet with me. On our last session together he came by himself on the long train journey and then by bus. We talked about his tremendous achievement and agreed that this was a new level of control and confidence in himself. This was an example of one incident whose significance would have been missed in the accepted approach to grief counselling. I found that in counselling people with aphasia, in particular, what seems to be a minor incident can be life changing.

5

Aphasia centres and community: more than just the sum of parts

Aura Kagan

Key points

- Aura works at the Aphasia Institute in Toronto, a community centre promoting conversation, social opportunity and participation in life.
- People living with aphasia are often encouraged to 'return to the community'.
- Aura thinks about what community means and how being part of different communities is important to feeling good about yourself.
- Community with a big 'C' refers to different sectors and roles in society: being a voter, a volunteer and a member of neighbourhood associations and community schemes.
- Community with a small 'c' refers to the groups that are part of our everyday lives: neighbours, church groups, friends and workmates.
- Aura thinks that people with aphasia often get cut off from both types of community.
- She talks about how it is possible to re-build communities with people who have aphasia, even if this is on a small scale.
- Sometimes this means re-connecting with old friends, interests and groups, but sometimes its about meeting new people and developing different friendships.

In this chapter I welcome the opportunity to reflect more deeply on an issue that has interested me for some time: namely, what it is that we really mean when we talk about 'community' in relation to aphasia and the services we provide? In terms of service, I am most familiar with those provided by the Aphasia Institute in Toronto, Canada where I have been involved since 1986. Let me begin by describing what first captured my imagination about this agency, and what has sustained an on-going interest and passion ever since.

I knew from the first day that I walked into the Aphasia Institute's Pat Arato Aphasia Centre (hereafter referred to as the Aphasia Centre), that I had stumbled upon something out of the ordinary in terms of services for people with aphasia. Prior to this, and after emigrating from South Africa, I had been working for a provincial home care service and had thus already been confronted with the reality of living with aphasia – a far cry from my previous therapy experience in university and hospital clinic rooms. However, nothing had prepared me for my first exposure to a room filled with several groups of people sitting around tables engaged in various activities. Some were using workbooks, others seemed absorbed in ordinary social interaction. Were these people the same as those with aphasia whom I had met in the course of my professional career up until that point? The extraordinary thing was that it all looked so ordinary. How was such engagement and interaction possible when many of these people had severe aphasia? I have spent much of my time since that first day trying to capture the essence of what made this experience so different.

I began with starting to describe the programmes of the Aphasia Centre as 'long-term' and 'community-based'. Up until that time there had been no formal acknowledgement of the fact that we wanted to move away from the idea that discharge from traditional therapy was the end of the line in terms of support. We wanted to introduce the idea that support needed to continue in the community. At that stage I thought of the term 'community-based' as meaning that our agency was physically situated in the community as opposed to a hospital or rehabilitation centre. This was reinforced by the involvement of professionally trained and supervised local community volunteers as deliverers of front-line service. For the past few years, however, I have been thinking about community in relation to aphasia and the service provided by the Aphasia Centre in a different sense.

For me the issue has come to the fore when trying to answer questions posed by others who want to start something like an aphasia centre but feel overwhelmed because of lack of resources, not knowing where to start. What is the kernel or core of what we do? The answers seem simple enough. For example, group work has been at the heart of our service from day one. We have also focused on training partners for individuals with aphasia, including volunteers, health professionals and family members. We will often advise therapists/clinicians interested in providing services to those living with aphasia to start with some of these activities.

However, enhancing access to a meaningful social fabric is bigger than providing group treatment or improving communication between a person with aphasia and a spouse. Although these are useful methods with sound underlying principles, they beg a bigger question related to their role in restoring a sense of community to those affected by aphasia. By the end of this chapter I hope to have moved forward in my thinking on the issue of 'community and aphasia'.

Reintegration into 'the community' is held out to be a primary goal of rehabilitation in aphasia therapy. But what exactly do we mean by 'the community'? I have learned from informal conversations with colleagues that we do not necessarily agree on this issue. Ways of judging the extent to which people participate in their community might include assessing whether or not they are active users of different community facilities, or whether they choose to vote or assume various community roles such as those of volunteers or leaders. I call community in this sense, the 'big C' Community. It is what is most visible and seems to be what most of us first think of when we hear the term 'community'.

Less commonly we might think of the 'small c' communities that we all participate in, and often take for granted. These might include a person's immediate family, extended family, work colleagues, different groups of friends, each with their own common bonds. For example, your community might include your school friends, those you have regular vacations with, special interest or hobby groups such as book groups, or communities related to religious activity. In contrast to 'the Community', these 'small c' communities are primarily based on interpersonal relationships. Both aspects of community are an intrinsic part of the social fabric of our lives and important to social well-being. How can we address the barriers imposed by aphasia in relation to this dual notion of community?

I will begin by teasing out examples of how centres such as the Aphasia Centre and others like it play a role in beginning to restore community to the lives of people with aphasia and their families. The goal is achieved through a combination of the following factors, rather than any one in isolation.

First, core activities take place in groups. Among the range of activities, there is always an emphasis on providing the opportunity to join groups for the express purpose of conversation, social interaction and interest, as opposed to focusing primarily on groups designed to restore language or compensate for communication problems. Group facilitators may be trained community volunteers, as is the case at the Aphasia Centre. Other centres use students or therapists, depending on needs and constraints. Importantly, these groups are accessible to anyone with aphasia, including those with very severe aphasia.

Second, the physical setting and atmosphere do not have the feel of a hospital or institution but rather of a vibrant adult community centre. The culture of the centre emphasizes caring, equality and involvement rather than being 'given care'. Thus, for example, people do not sit in a waiting room in readiness for a group leader to call them in for their activity. Group facilitators are encouraged *not* to take on the role of the 'expert' who chooses and manages activities and time with the goal of improving communication but, rather, to facilitate social interaction among group members. The skill of the facilitators lies in two main areas: knowledge of group process, and ability to provide appropriate conversational support. Facilitators are trained to ensure that group members know they are regarded as competent adults and to help them reveal this competence to each other within the group context.

Third, there is a critical mass of participants – not so many that it is overwhelming, but enough to allow for natural choice of social affiliation for both members and families. Individuals are able to exercise choice in both activities and social affiliation.

Fourth, all information, and the process of participation itself, is made as communicatively accessible as possible – what we call 'aphasia-friendly'. Information covers issues ranging from the personal (for example, letting people know what is happening to others in the community) to information about the organization (for example, issues to be discussed at the annual general meeting).

Finally, in addition to acquiring roles within a group, there is ample opportunity to participate and take on roles that extend beyond a specific group meeting time or activities within the Aphasia Centre. Opportunities normally available to adults are also made available within the broader Aphasia Institute, including the right to vote, to be eligible for membership on governing bodies, to take advantage of leadership opportunities and opportunities to be helpers as well as recipients of help. Equally important, people with aphasia can choose to do none of the above.

Thus, the kernel or core of what we provide may be the *choice* and *multiplicity* of community roles, relationships and small communities or groups that allow people to emerge as social beings. Without this, providing group therapy, training communication or conversation partners will not necessarily achieve the goal of restoring a sense of community to the lives of those affected by aphasia.

Let me illustrate with a few scenarios reflecting different degrees of participation in a community by members[1] of the Aphasia Institute. As with any of us entering a new organization, it often takes time for people to familiarize themselves with the way that things work, and to gain confidence. Following an initial period of acclimatization, which can take anything from a few weeks or months to a year or more, some members of the centre choose to expand their activities and/or involvement. Others choose to continue as they started and still others choose to leave and seek other possibilities. One wonders whether the latter include those who have retained at least some of their communities outside of the centres, or managed to create new ones themselves.

Pat

Recently Pat has chosen to participate in two conversation groups and an art class. He is a member of the Toronto Aphasia Advocacy Group as well as on the Advisory and Ethics Committee of the Aphasia Institute. In these groups he interacts with a variety of different people – in other words there is choice but also sufficient variety for this choice to be meaningful. He is clearly seeking involvement and, with increased confidence, is willing to take on more responsibility. Over time he has become comfortable with email. Although he cannot use it to sustain complicated dialogue, he does use email for practical purposes such as receiving notifications of events and reminding others of upcoming meeting dates. Pat has also started using computer software to help overcome his difficulties in reading text. The program 'reads aloud' scanned-in passages and he finds that this makes a big difference to his ability to comprehend text. One of his first actions is to let others know about this. He brings staff into the picture if he is talking to someone with more severe aphasia where he is not sure that the person is understanding him. A few other members have indicated interest and are pursuing use of this software. Pat makes full use of the range of opportunities offered by the Aphasia Centre – opportunities much like those any of us have in our communities.

Pat also has communities outside of the centre but these days this is mostly limited to his family. There is another really important 'small c' community for Pat within the Aphasia Institute. This comprises the people with whom he chooses to socialize outside of any of the formal activities of the centre. Social activities take place before and after the formal aspects of the programme, but are equally important. This community is diverse in every way, including people with varying severity of aphasia, but has *naturally* developed into a genuine community for its members. Recently Pat was unable to attend due to some health problems. However, his community kept in touch with him and were there when he was ready to return. Belonging to a community made a significant quality of life difference to him during this period of time. In other words, although Pat speaks frequently about the importance of maintaining and improving his communication, this is only a part of the story.

Pam

Pam volunteers in various capacities at the centre – in administration and in offering peer support. She has been at the centre for a long time, having suffered a stroke in her twenties. Pam's sense of humour and sarcastic wit are her trademark. Over the years I have noticed changes in her use of humour and sarcasm. Her ability to pick up on what others say in order to make fun of them has increased. In thinking about community I wonder whether having a ready community available to 'practise' humour, a community where mistakes are not interpreted as signs of incompetence, has been a factor in the development of Pam's use of humour. If she didn't have the centre, would she be able to use humour and sarcasm as part of an identity that she seems to enjoy?

Not everyone chooses to be as involved as Pat and Pam. Tom, for example, has come to a weekly drop-in club for years. He doesn't need to sign up for it or make any commitment but can just come when he chooses. Similarly, Don now also chooses to come once a week, but his activity of choice is an 'aphasia friendly' toastmasters' public speaking course. Fred built up his involvement in the centre over several years, topping it off with a stint as a member of the board of directors. Subsequently he became a volunteer for Meals on Wheels. When asked why he still came to the centre once a week he said, 'because of here, I can do that . . .' (meaning that his attendance at the centre gave him the confidence to pursue roles outside). At one time, he did stop coming but more recently has rejoined, needing support as he deals with a painful family situation.

Jila

Jila's spouse was committed to the idea of her regaining her language. He drove her and always waited while she participated in her activities. Jila is now confident enough to insist on using public transit and attending on her own because this is 'her' community. Most recently she has joined a committee of members in charge of putting out the internal publication for the Aphasia Institute.

Families and couples also form communities. For example, following our twelve-week introductory programme where strong bonds are formed, couples sometimes choose to continue meeting independently, either at home or in accessible restaurants. This is an example of community started because of the Aphasia Institute, but no longer occurring within its walls.

The option of long-term involvement is one of the important things about belonging to any community. However, when people with aphasia find a long-term community in an organization such as the Aphasia Centre, this is sometimes seen as a sign of dependence. Surely, if the intervention is working, we should see the results in people having the confidence to leave and function independently in real communities in the outside world? However, in my view the community and communities that people find within such a centre *are* real life – not a preparation for real life.

For me, this is not an either/or issue – one of special centres versus the real world – but rather one of choices. Many of our long-term members also participate in other communities such as church groups. However, they still feel the need for a community where aphasia is taken for granted and they don't even have to think about it. Reducing language barriers means that people with aphasia have increased communicative access to information and the 'system knowledge' that makes meaningful participation possible. In addition, opportunities to continue trying to improve communication is not that different to what many of us do in accessing community resources to help improve our skills in specific areas. Why should individuals with aphasia not have the right to this just as any of us can choose different participation options and contexts, some of which are more comfortable than others?

For me, the issue is less about justification of this principle than about logistics and funding. The challenge is to find a way to provide the type of long-term support that gives greater access to community in the sense described above so that it becomes an intrinsic part of best practice in the continuum of care.

In relation to the above, I wonder if our use of terminology makes a difference. As pointed out to us by a programme manager in our Ministry of Health, the idea of entitlement to long-term support for individuals with aphasia does not necessarily fit with the term 'rehabilitation'. In most people's minds rehabilitation has a finite end point. This arrives sooner in some systems and later in others, but rehabilitation is never on-going. People with chronic medical conditions or illnesses such as diabetes, however, receive on-going *treatment* rather than rehabilitation. In addition to the assumption that medical support in the form of insulin will be available forever, treatment consists of periodic check-ups to monitor health status and make adjustments to medications if necessary. In other words, treatment, unlike rehabilitation, does not necessarily imply improvement in the condition. It can include the goal of maintaining current status on the understanding that if such treatment were withdrawn, there would be serious consequences.

It is difficult to talk about the impact of withdrawal of the kind of support provided by centres such as ours, as relatively few people are served. However, based on my experience and that of my colleagues, I can tell you that services such as ours are often described as being a lifeline for those with aphasia and their families. The word 'treatment' does not fit easily into social model parlance because it is a medical term and is frequently used in relation to 'fixing' a condition. However, as with the example of people with diabetes, the term 'treatment' does not necessarily have to be used in this way. It may be worth thinking about whether or not it would be useful for us to get our healthcare systems to view interventions such as the long-term support provided by aphasia centres, as 'treatment'. The Aphasia Center of California has been doing this for some time.

A focus on restoring community to those affected by aphasia fits into the World Health Organization's acknowledgement of the importance of participation (World Health Organization 2001) and especially well into the values proposed by the Life Participation Approach to Aphasia (LPAA) (2001). Table 5.1 presents the potential role of aphasia centres in restoring community in relation to the values articulated by the LPAA. We have found it useful to be able to refer to these broad-ranging LPAA values as they capture our commitment to real life participation and the long-term needs of all those affected by aphasia.

At the beginning of this chapter, I mentioned the fact that we are constantly challenged to describe the essence of what we provide at the Aphasia Centre. It may be that centres such as ours have not been explicit enough about our potential role in restoring a sense of community in the two ways described in earlier sections. Thus, in answer to those who want to start a centre but only have the resources to start small, I would say that even if you are only able to begin with one group, and the setting is not ideal, you should endeavour to create to the greatest extent possible the factors that give a sense of belonging to a community. Examples may include offering choice and variety of social connection; opportunities for taking on different roles such as that of volunteer, committee member or leader; and opportunity to sustain long-term relationships and a sense of stability so that individuals can leave and have something to come back to as needed or desired.

On a more personal note, at the Aphasia Institute volunteers and staff also form communities. As with our members, the relatively large number of volunteers allows for formation of many small communities related to particular programmes and activities, and to factors such as starting at the same time and doing training together. The staff community too has its own unique culture that obviously includes but encompasses far more than commitment to a particular philosophy of professional practice. Features include awareness of the importance of interpersonal relationships that go beyond the workplace to incorporate support around family, other life issues and crises; and use of talents and passions wherever possible, rather than being required to fit a mould.

Table 5.1. Role of Aphasia Centres in restoring community as related to the values of the Life Participation Approach to Aphasia (LPAA)

LPAA Value	*Examples of potential role for Aphasia Centres*
1 Explicit goal is enhancement of life participation	Actually providing community (as opposed to preparing people for community) gives an explicit focus to life participation
2 All those affected by aphasia are entitled to service	Opportunity for individuals with aphasia, family members and/or couples to form natural small communities and participate in the larger community framework
3 Measures of success include documented life enhancement changes	Outcomes include documentation of participation within the Aphasia Centre community as well as outside of it
4 Personal and environmental factors are targets of intervention	Creating an environment where there are no communication barriers to full participation e.g. ensuring that all information is 'aphasia-friendly' and accessible to members. In the case of the Aphasia Institute, this would include items such as the vision and mission statement or issues to be voted on at the Annual General Meeting
5 Emphasis on availability of services as needed at all stages of aphasia	Aphasia Centres are in a unique position in terms of being able to fulfil this value and 'being there' for people with aphasia and their families as readiness for intervention, needs and life circumstances change

I mentioned earlier that I have spent much time thinking about how to capture the essence of what makes the Aphasia Centre so special. What captures my imagination and sustains an on-going interest and passion?

My answer to this question is rooted in my experience of 'community and communities' for everyone associated with the organization.

Note

1 Clients of the centre prefer being called 'members' – initially part of a deliberate attempt to distance themselves from medical terminology such as 'patients'. Membership in an organization also has a positive connotation.
   Members referred to by name have given me their permission to do so.

References

LPAA (Life Participation Approach to Aphasia) Project Group (2001) Life participation approach to aphasia: a statement of values, in R. Chapey (ed.) *Language Intervention Strategies in Aphasia and Related Neurogenic Communication Disorders.* Baltimore, MD: Lippincott, Williams and Wilkins.

World Health Organization (2001) *International Classification of Functioning, Disability and Health (ICF)* www.who.int/classification/icf

6

From doing to being: from participation to engagement

Alan Hewitt and Sally Byng

Key points

- Alan and Sally talk about their different experiences leading up to the time they started to work together.
- Alan reviews some of the things that happened to him after he had a brain haemorrhage. He describes shifting levels of engagement and involvement with family, friends, employers and organizations concerned with therapy and self-help.
- Sally reflects on the ways in which her thinking as a speech and language therapist has changed over years of work. For a long time she has wanted to find a way of working that would address the real life issues faced by people with aphasia and other communication impairments.
- Although their situations were very different, both Alan and Sally were striving for activities that were purposeful and meaningful, and relationships that were equal and mutually respectful.
- They have started to work together and with other people who have aphasia. Their first project focused on finding ways of involving people with aphasia in the running of a voluntary sector organization. This work has made them realize the power of engagement.
- The authors suggest that engagement (being and feeling valued) is different from participation (doing).
- While working towards the engagement of people with aphasia is not easy, it brings many benefits for everyone concerned.
- This work has made them think again about the purpose and nature of therapy for people with aphasia.

We wanted to write this chapter because we have come to recognize the potential impact of what we have called 'engagement', for people both with and without aphasia. We believe that this process of engagement could be used creatively to assist the process of learning to live life with aphasia, *and* to enable service providers to develop relevant services for people living with aphasia.

This chapter describes the journeys of two people who are working together as colleagues – one of us has aphasia, the other one doesn't. It describes the experiences that have motivated the work we are doing together now.

We will start by describing very briefly what we have felt to be the limitations of the current models of disability which underpin therapeutic work and service delivery, why we think engagement is different and why we feel excited by it. We will go on to tell our stories, which chart the routes we have taken to engagement, describe an experience of engagement, and finish by trying to define more clearly what we mean by the term and how we might recognize it.

Why 'engagement'?

So why are we fired up about engagement enough to want to write about it? For us, engagement offers a different way of thinking about both therapy for learning to live with aphasia and the collaborative development of services for people living with aphasia. In recent years the all encompassing medical model of healthcare has been challenged, and a social model, in various guises, has come to be more accepted as a basis from which to provide health and social services. We have seen the World Health Organization perspectives of 'impairment, disability and handicap' change into 'impairment, activity and participation', reflecting a new attitude towards people living with disabilities prompted by disability rights campaigners and theorists, enabling the location of disability outside of the individual.

However, we have found that even this shift in attitude leaves us with some unease. It assumes that the goals of people living with aphasia (or with any disability for that matter) all relate to 'doing', rather than to 'being'. It assumes that all people with disabilities want to participate and *do* things. The concepts of activity and participation have become interpreted by therapists as highlighting the importance of *function*, and the goals of much therapy are described these days as 'functional'. We appreciate acutely the importance of 'functioning' adequately. Doing (for yourself or for others), being active and participating, is vital for many people. It is necessary, but maybe not sufficient. Does 'doing' by itself necessarily make people feel more alive, to 'be' themselves? Our personal experiences separately made us feel that these concepts were not capturing satisfactorily what people need to connect with life with disability.

Recent experiences that we have both had of working together with people living with aphasia, in a way that felt different, have highlighted to us the idea that being 'engaged' is a critical component of learning to live with aphasia. We have begun to see the power of what we are describing as 'engagement' to enable people with aphasia to make changes not only in their lives, but also in their communication. So much therapy has as its goal the enhancement of communication in everyday life, but all therapists know the difficulties inherent in achieving this, and people with aphasia know its frustration. Yet we have seen people make substantial changes to the way they feel, communicate and relate to other people not as a result of what we might regard as conventional therapy, but as a result of becoming 'engaged' in different ways.

In this chapter we are trying to convey what we mean by 'engagement', how we have come to it and how we might facilitate more of it.

Routes to engagement

Our stories trace the origins of our involvement in our collaborative work, and provide the backdrop for what has influenced how we now work. We tell our stories independently, before coming together to describe the work which we interpret as 'doing engagement'. Alan Hewitt sees his evolving life with aphasia as a series of doors which he has opened or which have opened for him. Sally Byng sees her working life as a series of windows she has looked through, each giving her a new perspective on her quest – to provide better services for people learning to live with aphasia. So we describe the various doors and windows we experienced until we both reached the 'same room' and started to work collaboratively. Then we will briefly describe a project that we have been involved in together. From this experience we will extrapolate what we mean by engagement and how we see its potential for those of us involved in learning to live with aphasia.

Alan Hewitt: doors to engagement

I'd just taken my two daughters home from my girlfriend Anne's house, in 1992. I had been seeing Anne for about three months, and we were just getting to know each other. I suddenly had this *gigantic, splitting* headache. Apparently an aneurysm in the cerebral artery had split the artery and was seeping blood into my brain. My brain was scanned and operated on.

The surgeon 'clipped' my left cerebral artery in my head, where it had split causing a subarachnoid haemorrhage.

Of all problems that I had to deal with – having no speech, no movement on the right side – the social isolation was profound. Most of my friends from before the brain haemorrhage faded away, apart from a few. Most of them came to see me in hospital, or just after I had left the hospital, and then went their own way. I was just a person with no speech and no language at all, and if I didn't have that kind of speaking/ communication relationship, that relationship where I was a *whole* person. All that which was so important, in retrospect, was swept aside into the dustbin. All that mattered to me was just screwed up and thrown away. The questions where was I, who was I, and what on earth was a whole person, were more pertinent than I could guess.

My daughters, Joanna and Jess, helped me, though they didn't know it. Just seeing them there 'fortified' me. I know that seeing me there, wrapped up in intensive care, was a shock for them. I feel that one of the reasons I pulled through it was because of the love I felt for them, and their love for me. I didn't want them to say 'that's the last I saw of my dad, cocooned up in intensive care with bits of him wired up to machines'.

My relationship with my girlfriend, Anne, dwindled away over the six months or so after the brain haemorrhage. Looking back, I can feel myself standing in the doorway of that flat and waving goodbye to Anne, as she drove away. And feeling relieved. I was on my own.

Speech and language therapy . . . of sorts

It was about two years after my haemorrhage that I began to make 'progress' in language. Just once a week I'd toddle off to get my 'therapy fix'. I had speech and language therapy for about two and a half years to three years. At that time there was no sign of a charity to help me . . . for me to realize that what I'd got was a disability called aphasia, not just some freakish whim of nature, was very important to me. It has to do with the place where I was, and who I was, and how I tried to communicate. I was *waiting* for *anyone* opening doors to 'real social engagement'. I realize now I was just waiting. It takes two to tango.

Door no 1 . . .

Before my haemorrhage I was a manager at a fuel poverty charity. The charity kept me on when I was ready to get back to work, in a justifiably downgraded job, as an information officer. They probably didn't know what to do with me, but they stuck by me. I got a computer at work and learnt very slowly what to do with it.

As I got better with language, I looked through the papers for press cuttings for the organization. I spotted one day a piece in the newspaper that was about dysphasia. Reading it through slowly I realized *I had dysphasia*, or *aphasia*, and the address of the charity to write to!

I wrote a letter to Action for Dysphasic Adults (ADA, now Speakability) a charity for people with aphasia whose address I *now* knew, and the whole thing rolls on from there. I went to London for an introductory session, got in touch with Carol Wisdom, an ADA Regional Development Officer, set up with Carol and my speech language therapist a session for people in my Gateshead community who had aphasia to set a group going. I got the ADA Gateshead self-help group established. I became the Secretary. It was hard work but I did it, with Carol's help.

I felt more of a *place* in the social scheme of things. I felt more *self-esteem* as a person. Having a place in a self-help group to help people with aphasia, as the secretary, I felt more *grounded* than just a 'has-been'. I was 're-engaging' with life.

Door no 2 . . .

Now I was into the swing of things (as far as it can be when you've got aphasia) I went down to London for meetings of the ADA Regional Committee for self-help groups.

At one of the meetings I met Cressida Laywood, of Aphasia Nottingham, and before I knew it I was moving in with her. That was in 1997 – now I am Secretary of Aphasia Nottingham and she is the Chair.

I left my job. I 'left' my two daughters – although I still keep in touch with them, seeing them once a month. I left the self-help group for people with aphasia I had set up. I left my old life behind. I said hello to Nottingham and to Cressida. Unfortunately, when you are trying to achieve engagement in life, you have to take the rough times with the smooth.

Cressida and I went to Canada and America in 2000 for seven aphasia lectures. That's quite an art in itself, the two of us, two people with aphasia, let loose on the US and Canada. It was the *two of us* doing what we *cared* about, and doing it *together*. But there's a downside to this. We lacked the professional and 'academic' engagement to go that little bit further with our trip on our return. We had a bit of funding, but that was the limit of our professional backing. We had the trip's PowerPoint computer lectures ready to go. We gave talks to four aphasia groups, and the Nottingham speech and language therapists – but that's all. It could have been built on professionally – how could we have got professionals to engage with us and what we had to say?

However, I have a lot to be grateful to aphasia for:

- I have made *new friends* – all to do with aphasia.
- I have confronted *new challenges and opportunities* – all to do with aphasia.
- I have made *new ideas and concepts* – all to do with aphasia.

All of these things have to do with getting engaged in a new life.

Door no 3 . . .

I felt that when I was receiving speech and language therapy at first, nothing much made any sense. There was too much to do, along with the physical therapy I was going through. I had 'homework' to do, and I religiously followed it. I remember thinking 'this speech and language therapy is *not* working for me'. I just went there and did that. I just wanted something more. I just wanted a sense of *social engagement*. I wanted a *social* context, not just the random *health* context that the National Health Service gave me.

The sense of engagement was to find a place where what I did had a relevance to people with aphasia, and to me. Some overall structure that I could relate to . . . it may have to do with the charity development work I did before, but perhaps more to do with me.

When I had a structure I could fit with, like the self-help groups coupled into ADA, it was easier to do. It was a social set of circumstances. It was *real* to me. I could see what you could put in and what you could get out. I wanted to get into the national structure of ADA (Speakability). I was elected Vice-chair of the ADA Regional Committee of self-help groups (I was going to be Chair). I was appointed to the editorial board of *Speaking Up*, the Speakability journal. I had a sense of going forward, inch by inch.

Door no 4 . . .

Then out of the blue I got a letter from Sally Byng, Chief Executive at Connect (then a new communication disability, not-for-profit organization), asking me to be a member of the Board of Trustees for Connect. I jumped at it and accepted because I knew the group and liked their work. Dynamite. I resigned from the Speakability posts.

That was in 2000. Since then I have been placed with making sure the people with aphasia *have a voice* in the charity, and in the charity's structure. I did this as a trustee to begin with, and then in 2002 I got a salaried job in Connect as Working Together Co-ordinator – still with the task of working out how people with aphasia can be involved in shaping the organization.

I wouldn't want anyone to think it has been easy, getting 'engaged' with life. All along the line I have gone down side alleys, gone the wrong way, ended up shored in dead end streets, in some ways looking for 'engagement'. But I kept going because that is the way I felt alive. No matter if I can't feel the way I did, if I can't speak the way I did, can't remember the way I did, can't play the guitar *at all* – that's the way it is. But engagement, that is about *people*, getting through to each other, which is all to me.

Door no 5 . . . a true sense of engagement

There's a real sense of true social and self-engagement in me, if I can just pry it apart – it has perhaps to do with:

- *Communicating* with a *realistic social target* to reach with people with aphasia. Then when it's hit, try the *next* social target, and *reflecting*.
- *Coming to realize* that perhaps it's the people with aphasia who are after a sense of true engagement in the *real* and *concrete* social world.
- *Connecting*, through Connect and Aphasia Nottingham, with people with aphasia and professionals who just want to communicate. Just people!

Looking through windows: Sally Byng's story so far

My first window, through which I viewed therapy and engaged with people with communication disabilities, was the first therapy room that I worked in. The sign on the door said 'Speech and language therapist'. It grew to unnerve me. Didn't 'therapist' mean that I was supposed to know how to make someone better? But what did 'better' mean for the people I was working with? And what was the therapy that would help them achieve that?

I worked with young people who had had head injuries. Complex problems at a complex time in people's lives. Every day I faced people whose lives had turned upside down. The people I saw either couldn't speak, or I couldn't follow what they said. Often they couldn't walk, dress or eat either. They might not know where they were, who they were, who their families were or who I was. These things meant that life as they had lived it was no longer possible for them or, for that matter, for their families.

What did I do? To begin with I turned to my professional armoury – I got out my course notes, I read articles, I tried to match up some of the issues I was facing with text books I got from the library. The problem was, nothing that I read seemed to relate to what I thought I needed to do. I thought I needed to figure out what was wrong with someone and do something about it. The trouble was I wasn't happy with the interpretations I could reach of what was 'wrong'. I turned to another part of the therapist's armoury – tests and assessments – for points of reference in the fog that surrounded me. Standardized language tests. They showed up what someone could and couldn't do in relation to language and speech. That helped – but didn't tell me *why* they had difficulty. Or what to do. Or what was really 'wrong' in the big picture of their lives.

I think I really wanted to engage with that big picture, but I didn't know where to begin. There seemed to be a chasm between what I 'knew' from the tests I carried out and what I could imagine when I thought about the immensity of the problems that a person faced. I simply didn't understand enough.

I was rescued by research. A window tinted by rationalism. I thought let's understand *why* someone has the communication problem that they have and then I might understand more what to do about it. And if I keep the problem I am trying to understand contained, then it will be less overwhelming to try to unpick. I felt much better for a while. I could tell myself that if I understood more about the problem, then I could provide more rationally motivated therapy. Creating principled order in what felt to me like therapy chaos.

And I did. Furthermore I could demonstrate the effects of therapy scientifically. This took me so far, but then I realized what was probably already evident to others before. The kind of therapy that I was doing, even though it was rational, principled and could change some aspects of someone's language, was not making any significant difference to some-one's ability to live their changed life as a changed person. Yes, language and speech could change, and we could show that it was therapy that could contribute to bringing about that change. But how did that relate to helping someone to turn their world less upside down?

I perceived acutely a credibility gap in what I was doing. Perhaps I was feeling the therapist's equivalent of what Alan felt about his therapy: where was the social engagement, the communicating with a realistic social target? Where was the connection to *life* and what someone just wanted to *be*? I didn't find the movement at that time in speech and language therapy towards 'functional' therapy any more reassuring either. Although it seemed to be about every day life, for me it offered only a very specific perspective on real life – about doing practical things rather than being a person. Of course there is a relationship between doing and how you feel about yourself – but the doing seemed to be so basic that I couldn't see how to make the leap from that to re-connecting with life again as a different person.

The rescuers were not in sight this time. I spent a long time looking for another window – another way of doing therapies that connected with this bigger picture. Perhaps instead of trying to understand the problem I could try another tack in my drive to bring some kind of rationalism and logic for myself in doing therapy. What I thought was this. Therapists do therapy and often it seems to 'work'. Perhaps if I understood how the therapy worked I could feel better about doing it and do it more effectively. I can imagine what you are thinking: in hindsight it doesn't seem the logical way to go about trying to work out how to address a spinning world for people facing massive personal change. But the complexity of that spinning world seemed overwhelming. I was trying to be logical about what I was doing as a therapist, understand it and be rational about it. How could I be rational about upside down worlds?

I did finally find another window on what I was doing. This time it was understanding more about the process of doing language therapy. The therapy I was trying to do aimed to enable someone with aphasia to have greater control over their own language and communication for themselves. It was exciting in a way that I hadn't found in therapy before.

I had always found therapy sessions stimulating and intriguing – never routine. However, I think this was for me my first taste of what felt like real engagement in therapy: shared understanding of the complexities of what we were doing, a shared spirit of trying to solve problems and dilemmas about language and communication together. But the dilemmas and problems were still very small in scale (if not in linguistic complexity). I was still unnerved by their lack of connection to the day-to-day issues of people living with aphasia. Their lack of connection to engagement in life.

I could rationalize to myself that the better the control someone had over their language and communication, then the better prepared they would be to engage in life. So it was profitable to work specifically on language and communication skills. I still believe that to be true. But only if we are at the *same time* supporting people to deal with the multiplicity of other issues that they are grappling with in their changed worlds, which are often more overwhelming – to the person living with them as well as to the therapist.

The prompt for my fourth window, which has provided a perspective for me for the last ten years, was provided by Oliver (1992):

Researchers have benefitted by taking the experience of disability, rendering a faithful account of it and then moving to better things while the disabled subjects remain in exactly the same social situation they did before the research began.

When I read this all too uncomfortably accurate description of my own working life, I realized that I could no longer avoid those changed worlds. If I was to retain any connection to the word therapist then I had to start thinking about how to be rational about supporting people in dealing with their changed communication in the context of the complexities of their lives.

By this time I was engaging with therapy at second hand – as a researcher/teacher/colleague. I found it safer at a distance – cowardly perhaps, but authentic to how I was feeling. I became a commentator. I listened to people's stories – people living with communication disabilities, people researching and people providing therapy. I tried to make sense of it all – to see how the pieces of the bigger jigsaw fitted together. What really mattered to people whose lives had changed? What were the issues for therapists? What concerned researchers? How did they relate to each other to come together for the benefit of people living with aphasia?

The window I was then beginning to look through had a very different view from the previous ones, but parts of it were still recognizable. I could see where what I had done before fitted in, but now the view was much bigger. My colleagues were helping me to see some routes in to supporting changed lives. I didn't feel skilled enough to know how to follow those routes myself, but I could begin to understand them, see how they could work and try to describe them with other people.

That has taken me to the window I'm looking through now. With my colleagues I have established a new service for people living with aphasia, called Connect – the communication disability network, outside of the usual health systems in the UK. It is a not-for-profit organization, promoting innovative therapy and support services that focus on enabling people living with aphasia to re-engage with life with aphasia. At Connect we work with people to re-think communication, identity and lifestyle with aphasia. It is hard – not straightforward. We don't achieve what many people want – to have their communication back the way it was. But I can see that what we do achieve is to enable many people to cope more easily with the complexities, uncertainties and difficulties of living with aphasia, and being a person with aphasia, as well as enhancing communication skills.

What I am doing now is learning to work collaboratively, engaging differently with people with aphasia, in the role of a colleague with expertise, not as an expert – for me a crucial difference. What I mean by this is that I see that the skills and knowledge that I have acquired in my role as a professional enable me to have something useful to offer to people with aphasia. But my professional skills and knowledge do not give me a privileged position. They give me a basis from which to negotiate, discuss and share my perceptions to see how they fit with those of the person living with aphasia. Depending on the issue we are discussing I may or may not have more knowledge and expertise, and I feel free to make this clear. The point is that I am trying to combine my knowledge and skills with those of people with aphasia, which are of equal value, to find constructive ways of working together, making decisions and moving forwards. This feels for me like a very different way of engaging both with people living with aphasia, with whom I have a working relationship, and with users of our services. I am beginning to understand the impact and implications of these different relationships for developing services, which for me has been a liberating, creative and enlightening experience.

Working together and feeling engaged, the Having a Voice project

We have so far described independently the different doors and windows we have walked and looked through to reach this point. Now we describe together some joint work that we have undertaken which has helped us to see how we as people with and without aphasia can work together to promote 'engagement'. We have come to see engagement as a critical part not only of the therapeutic process, but also of the relationship between provider and user of services. As an example of what we mean, we will briefly describe a project that we have undertaken together, the Having a Voice project.

With the aim of providing ways for people who have aphasia to have a voice in the workings of our organization, we created a working party that would put proposals to the Board of Trustees at Connect about how people with aphasia could influence the way the organization is developing and could feed back on the quality and range of services. Our project had several stages: planning, meeting as a working party, creating a report and evaluating the process.

Planning

We first needed to find people with aphasia who were interested in serving on the working party. We (Alan) informed them of the party by designing an accessible PowerPoint slide show that was presented to different therapy groups at Connect. Ten people volunteered, some with no speech or writing, or with some difficulty understanding, and the group began to meet. We put communication support in place to ensure that all working party members could get their message across and understand each other.

Meeting

For each meeting, we created an agenda and selected supporting pictures/agendas/minutes to make sure the ideas being discussed would be accessible.

Discussions during the meetings revolved around the following issues:

- how to achieve authentic involvement from those with aphasia in the business of the organization;
- whether our goal was to create a user-led or user-sensitive organization;
- how to create representation for people with aphasia on Connect's Board of Trustees.

Evaluating and writing up the outcome

A final report was drafted by Alan, the Chair of the working party, then reviewed by a small group of people with aphasia, and finally agreed upon by the whole of the working party. It was submitted to the Trustees.

We asked people with aphasia what they thought about the working group. They made the following kinds of comments: 'interesting'; 'Brilliant ... friends ... bantering'; 'I [indicated "valued"] ... the enthusiasm and the contribution of people who can't speak'; and 'For any group of people with aphasia – top of the musts – ground rules'.

Their responses suggest that the group provided a feeling of engagement not only for us but for all participants. Their sense of engagement and what they got from the group was expressed in different ways. They described feelings of friendship, rapport, understanding of other people's communication difficulties, insight into how to work together and making a contribution to something real.

Engagement in this project meant different things to each of us. But our common feeling was that we felt engaged because the project felt 'real'. It involved real goals and the group members' input was genuinely significant. It also felt real because its outcome was of lasting importance to the organization. For example, the project has:

- enabled us to think more clearly about realistic ways of involving people with aphasia;
- given us confidence about our ability to develop our services effectively and in a way that is relevant to people living with aphasia;
- also given us confidence about the future of our decision-making processes;
- provided us with a way of ensuring mutual engagement in our future with our key group of stakeholders;
- given us the awareness and experience of real engagement.

We think that the project felt real to all the working party participants because it allowed people to express their feelings, thoughts, frustrations and hopes and because their input made a difference in the concrete world. It made people a crucial part of solving a problem.

Engagement and involvement in this project was hard work: hard work for the non-aphasic people involved, such as the communication supporter, and also for the people with aphasia. It was hard work because it dealt with the *whole person* and not just a person with aphasia.

So what do we mean by 'engagement'?

What is interesting to us is that this sense of engagement came from a group which was not a conventional therapy group. People with aphasia often comment that they get this sense of friendship, rapport, under-standing of other people's communication difficulties, and insight into how to work together from going to a wide range of therapy and self-help groups – the literature on group therapy attests to this. What is interesting for us was that this group did not purport to be a therapy or support group in any way, and yet people seemed to find it therapeutic. It was a way of being themselves, a concrete way. We have noticed that in other activities where we work collaboratively with people with aphasia as advisers, trainers and collaborators this same sense of 'therapeutic engagement' emerges.

What we have wanted to do in this chapter therefore is to provide a label, an identity, for what is happening in many of the therapy contexts that people are now developing around the world. We sense a general movement away from seeing therapy as an opportunity just to learn to *do* things, towards creating opportunities where people living with aphasia can *be* and *feel* valued, and in so doing find a way of connecting their new day-to-day lives with who they are (or want to be) as people. This is therapy as engagement, not just participation, in life.

A spin-off from this work is that we have noticed that people with aphasia often communicate and talk better during and after participating in engagement experiences. Although we have had a tendency to play this observation down up until now (as we would never have claimed that this was a potential side-effect of this work), we no longer feel we can ignore that some people can make considerable communicative gains through purposeful involvement and engagement. These gains are of the sort that we would have expected to happen through direct therapy for communication, and which often seem so elusive and difficult to achieve.

The experience of engagement for us has a range of characteristics:

- being involved in something which has real purpose, feels personally meaningful and valuable;
- being involved reciprocally – all parties getting something out of being or working together;
- providing a sense of real connection to other people with whom you can identify – getting through about real things;

- sharing an understanding of the issues that you are trying to address, or the solving of a problem with communicating in a real life context about real life things;
- providing a meaningful structure to enable you to connect with life;
- confronting real challenges;
- seizing opportunities;
- being involved companionably and respectfully.

This is challenging us to:

- extend our concepts of what 'therapy' means; and
- broaden our understanding of what 'therapy' services might offer in order to enable people to reconnect with life.

Perhaps the concept of therapy could be extended to incorporate authentic inclusion, partnership and engagement. If, in doing this, people living with aphasia can be involved in consultation and planning about services to be provided, therapists and people with aphasia could be in a 'win-win' situation: developing relevant and effective services at the same time as providing development opportunities for therapists and people with aphasia alike.

Reference

Oliver, M. (1992) Changing the social relations of research production? *Disability, Handicap and Society*, 7(2): 101–14.

7

Do I have green hair? 'Conversations' in aphasia therapy

Leanne Togher

Key points

- Leanne is interested in the types of conversations that take place between people with and without aphasia.
- In this chapter she reflects on some of the 'odd' things and strange activities a speech and language therapist may ask a client to do.
- Speech and language therapists often try to find out what difficulties a person with aphasia is having in communication by asking them to describe pictures or say the names of objects.
- She thinks people with aphasia may find these activities alarming and off-putting.
- Leanne thinks that these activities don't really say much about how the person is managing in day-to-day life.
- She suggests ways in which a therapist can get a better idea of day-to-day communication, by sharing experiences and having more natural conversations.

Imagine you are 55 years old and sitting out on your back patio with someone who knows you well, someone whom you have known for nearly 40 years. Maybe you studied together, travelled overseas together and raised your children at the same time. There have been years of sharing good times, joking around and also getting through difficult times. Imagine having a chat with that person. While having a coffee you might be talking about the weekend that is coming up. There is a dinner you are both going to with some of your friends and everyone is bringing a different dish. So you might talk about what you are both planning to take, who else will be there and you might even have a bit of a gossip about one of the group who seems to be having a mid-life crisis. You might show your friend some new photos and your friend might give her opinion about a world event that she heard about on the radio on the way to your place. Asking for advice, recounting interesting events, providing opinions and talking about feelings, frustrations and expectations are all part of what we would consider to be a conversation.

Of course, we don't just have conversations with friends. We also have conversations with people whom we do not know, quite successfully. For example, think about the dinner party where you meet someone new or the casual conversation you have with someone on the bus on the way home. We have different conversations according to how well we know our communication partner, and we seem to be able to adapt to these differences without even thinking about it.

Now let us move to an aphasia therapy session. As a 55-year-old woman you have had a stroke with a moderate aphasia so that your speech is halting and difficult. You manage to get out some key words, but it helps if your communication partner asks questions where they give you a choice of answers, or refer to something concrete such as photos. You are seated at a table in a small room which has a Monet picture on the wall, a notice board covered with pieces of paper that you cannot read and a desk covered with files and workbooks. You are facing a young woman who looks like she is in her early twenties. She appears to be very busy as she organizes papers, sets up a pile of objects, gets out a stopwatch and puts a tape in the tape recorder on the table in front of you. You wonder what on earth she is going to do with the objects – a ball, a replica gun, a hammer – and you are feeling a bit nervous about the tape recorder. After all, you have never really been recorded before, and now you can hardly speak you are being asked to talk into a microphone.

As the session progresses you wait at each step for the young woman to tell you what to do next. 'Tell me what happened to you? Tell me about this picture.' Well you can hardly see the picture – is that a boy with a kite and why are those people picnicking in their own front yard? 'Point to the cup, show me the arrow, is your name Smith? Read this sentence and do what is says – gloze you ears – what does that mean? Write your name, the alphabet, copy out this sentence' (which really makes no sense at all). She asks a number of other questions to which you have to answer yes or no: 'Do I have green hair?' Clearly she doesn't have green hair – what a question! The young woman seems satisfied enough as she packs away the objects and the pictures. Thank heavens for that. You ask when the session will be finished. She looks up at you and says 'We're nearly finished. So what are you planning for the weekend?' You manage to get out the words: 'Out . . . Dinner . . . friends.' The young woman says, 'Oh so you are having dinner with friends – tell me about that.' Oh this is going to be difficult. This person doesn't know any of your friends, your history with them, and why does she need to know anyway? Does this have some influence on what she is going to do in the next session? You manage to get out: 'old friends . . . bring food'. And for five long minutes, the young woman asks questions about what you've just said. You ask again if the session can end soon. Finally, the session comes to an end and you are feeling quite exhausted. Do you feel like you've had a conversation? Probably not.

Now put yourself in the place of the aphasia therapist. You have a 45-minute session to evaluate Mrs X, a 55-year-old woman who has had a left-sided stroke. You have a total of five sessions to assess her and provide some treatment. You want to get a baseline on key language modalities, her naming skills, her ability to produce a picture description, read, write, her auditory comprehension skills and have her produce some conversation at the end. All in all you think that the session went quite well. Mrs X was basically cooperative, a bit slow to respond and conversation was obviously very difficult for her. You doubt that she would manage a conversation with her friends or family. Clearly she had problems initiating ideas and presented with a moderate non-fluent aphasia. You plan next session to do some more work on investigating her semantic skills and see about organizing a communication book to help her in conversation. She might need extra encouragement to be involved in conversation as that is where she became a bit uncooperative. You ask Mrs X's husband for some photos of family members before they leave.

This scenario is not uncommon in aphasia therapy around the world. There is some recognition in the above sequence that language needed to be assessed above the level of the sentence or clause. This therapist included a warm-up interview, a picture description and a brief section at the end termed 'conversation'. Unfortunately these are often the only concessions made to evaluating the person's 'functional' communication. Aphasia therapists frequently make judgements based on these brief snippets of data that will determine the person's treatment goals and influence the way the person with aphasia views their new way of communicating. This chapter will argue that a great deal of information can be gleaned from some of the standard procedures in assessment for aphasia therapy, depending on the way this information is interpreted. Specifically, sociolinguistic methods of inquiry can complement the more traditional ways of viewing spoken texts produced in the therapeutic setting. But more importantly, it is argued that the interactions that occur in a therapy room are representative of a separate and distinct context which does not tell us about a person's conversation skills with their friends and family. To gain insight into a person's communication in their real world we need to take a step outside traditional methods. This chapter will provide some suggestions regarding how to do this.

Historical perspectives

Aphasia is essentially an impairment affecting a person's access to and use of language processes. Aphasia compromises a person's ability to communicate in daily life activities. The most noticeable manifestations of this impairment may include a difficulty finding words, putting sentences together, understanding what is said, reading, writing, telling the time and making calculations. It is no surprise then that early proponents who worked in the area of describing aphasia focused on language tasks at the word and sentence level. This tradition has continued into the present day, with the development of a range of sophisticated ways to evaluate the breakdown in underlying language processes that produce aphasia. These advances, based on cognitive neuropsychological processes, have provided a welcome and necessary addition to the practice of aphasia therapy.

In concert with these advances throughout the 1980s and 1990s came the emergence of discourse analysis as a therapy tool. Aphasia therapists became increasingly aware of the importance of examining the connected speech of the individual, leading to the use of assessment materials to elicit genres or discourse types such as narrative, procedural, expository (or giving an opinion) and so-called conversational texts. These different discourse types are evaluated because they have different purposes and require different language resources. For example, a narrative, which involves telling a story, typically has an introduction, a complicating action, a resolution and a final comment or summary (which is also known as a coda). In contrast, a procedural text, which describes how to do something such as describing the way to the train station, uses different types of language to a narrative and involves a series of instructional steps. An expository text is where the person is asked to give their opinion about a topic, such as their point of view on smoking in public places. Here, the text will describe a point of view, supported by a number of arguments. Finally, conversation, in the truest sense, describes a two-way interaction where people exchange ideas, introduce different topics and take turns in an equal way. The problem is, however, that what aphasia therapists describe as 'conversation' in their reports usually come about as the result of a structured interview. As Simmons-Mackie (2000: 166) suggested, a problem is the way 'spontaneous communication' is measured by many aphasia therapists. Traditional methods target isolated linguistic elements such as number of content words or grammatical completeness. These fail to examine the 'social devices and strategies that help us craft social interaction'. Before examining the features of 'conversations' within a therapeutic context, it may be useful to think about the characteristics of conversations in other contexts, with a view to differentiating why these are essentially very different.

What is conversation?

As can be seen from the example at the beginning of this chapter, there are hallmark features to conversation. Typically, a conversation between familiar participants has the following features.

It is part of a 'macro-conversation' (one that continues from one occasion to the next). It is structured according to the familiarity and relative status of the participants. It may have a number of sub-genres, such as recounts and expository sections. That is, a conversation can have a number of embedded sections, where people may tell stories that they have just remembered, or give an opinion about something their communication partner has introduced. The term 'conversation' can therefore encompass other discourse types, and is not simply the exchange of ideas or a series of topic progressions. The structure of conversation can therefore be quite complex. It may be recursive, in that topics will re-arise either within that particular conversation or over a number of different instances of conversations. Finally, both participants in the conversation have equal opportunity to contribute to the unfolding social process that is occurring.

Conversation is a much discussed phenomenon across a range of disciplines, including anthropology and linguistics, and has even been described as the basis for producing art. Modjeska (1999: 141), in her eloquent account of the life of Australian artist Stella Bowen, described the notion of conversation as a 'way of talking that comes with the breaking of formalities within families and between men and women, that comes with the intense inquiry into the drama of self and consciousness'. Modjeska (1999) describes the importance of conversation in the development of Stella's art, with an acknowledgement that:

conversation was for her the basis for intimacy: the real exchange that occurs between people who are open to each other in feeling and ideas. That kind of exchange, that kind of talk, mattered in the way she lived her life day to day, and in the way she came to understand herself.

Stella Bowen used this knowledge to paint people in conversation. *Provençal Conversation*, a painting in which she depicts two men and two women sitting in a French garden, captures the intimacy of the participants who are pausing in their discourse but appear completely relaxed and comfortable to simply be together. It is this notion of conversation that underlies the first example in this chapter of two friends catching up with each other, and that rarely occurs in the clinic room.

When we have a conversation, we are coding our own reality linguistically. That is, we use conversation to construct and organize the social situation by 'providing a foundation for personal relations and the socialization process, maintaining and giving a history of personal identity and creating and modifying the structure of reality' (Halliday 1994: 10). With increased familiarity, as with our first example, much of the foundation for personal relations is laid, as is the history of our personal identity. Conversation therefore serves to develop and maintain this history and create new realities within the background knowledge of who both participants are and their shared knowledge. When strangers interact, such as when people strike up a conversation at the bus stop, they may spend little energy on developing a history of personal identity, but they will be creating a new reality.

'Conversations' in the aphasia therapy assessment

'Conversation' is frequently seen as a warm-up task before the 'true' therapy commences, or as a way of wrapping up the session. So what is happening during this period when a therapist has a 'conversation' with the client? Silvast (1991) described the typical conversation with people who have aphasia as follows: 'The therapist makes a request for information, aphasic responds, often with an extended answer, and therapist follows with short answers' (1991: 388). Aphasia therapists rarely maintain and give a history of their own personal identity. In fact, it is sometimes thought to be unprofessional if one exposes too much personal information to one's clients. The on-going reality of the development of conversation from one session to the next is also arbitrary and artificial. The inherent power imbalance between the therapist and the client means that the therapist will usually introduce the topics to be discussed which frequently centre around completion of practice, attendance at other groups or therapy activities and social events. The macro-genre of conversation from one session to the next will usually concern these client-focused types of topics. The client is usually a passive recipient in this process (Parr 1996; Kovarsky *et al.* 1999). There is little reciprocity of linguistic options here as the client is unable to question the therapist, except perhaps to ask if they are busy or did they have a nice lunch. It would be considered inappropriate by some therapists for a client to ask whether they had attended other activities through the week, or to inquire about their weekend. There are also subtle rules and boundaries as to which type of genres a client can initiate. A phone call from a client to a therapist needs to have a purpose – changing an appointment or updating therapy progress, for example. It would be considered strange for a client to simply ring up for a chat.

This discussion may appear to be somewhat of a criticism of aphasia therapy practice, however, there are two important arguments which arise:

1 The activities described in a typical assessment interaction can be reframed sociolinguistically, rather than using traditional measurement techniques, and therefore be eminently more useful to the therapist. This begs the question of how a traditional aphasia assessment might be reframed sociolinguistically.
2 The notion of linguistic choice is important. Rather than 'choosing' to have linguistic power in an interaction this is usually unconscious and to a certain extent predetermined by the context, particularly the speaking situation (for example, a therapy interaction) and who is involved (for example, people with aphasia and therapists). The next step in this realization is to ask whether we need to address this imbalance. If we do, how do we do this?

How can a traditional aphasia assessment be reframed sociolinguistically?

Think back to our example where Mrs X is undergoing a therapy assessment. Traditionally, this could be represented as:

1 Brief warm-up – record Mrs X's responses and derive a count of mean length of utterance (MLU).
2 Standardized assessment (Western Aphasia Battery) – produce an Aphasia Quotient score.
3 Conversation at the end: measure MLU, measure ratio of nouns and verbs.

By evaluating these data using sociolinguistic resources, a much richer interpretation can be made of this same information. The discipline of sociolinguistics is concerned with language in its social context. It is interested in 'why we speak differently in different social contexts ... and identifying the social functions of language and the ways it is used to convey social meaning' (Holmes 1992: 1). So, in studying the way the interactions unfolded in Mrs X's initial assessment session, we would be implicitly aware that both the therapist and Mrs X jointly produced spoken texts which were specific to their therapist–client roles, and that their language enacted these roles. With this knowledge, the texts could be analysed using some of the many perspectives that are drawn from sociolinguistics (Armstrong 1992, 2000; Ferguson 1994; Togher 2001). For example, rather than simply scoring the length and number of Mrs X's utterances, the warm-up could be evaluated by looking at the range of speech functions Mrs X engaged in (for example, confirming, checking, clarifying, refuting). Of particular interest would be the variety of words Mrs X used as she recounted her story, for example, the range of verbs used perhaps comparing those denoting action (I *fell* down; couldn't *walk*) with those which help in describing feelings (I *was* scared; frightened, I *felt* awful), or other words which tell us about whether she can report what others have said (She *said* I had a stroke) or whether she can report verbal occurrences (I *called* out; I *spoke*). The nature of the stages or generic steps used in her story could be described using the generic stages of a recount (orientation which involves an introduction of who is involved, where the story occurs, a record of events and a coda or summary at the end). Her ability to assist in the repair of communication breakdown could also be gauged, for example, her use of verbal and nonverbal strategies, appeals for help to the therapist and willingness/ability to respond to strategies such as guessing attempts by the therapist. From making these types of analyses, and being aware of the limits of any conclusions that can be made because of the limited context, the therapist will have a much more detailed view of Mrs X's strengths within the assessment setting.

Another option is for therapists to rely less on standardized measures and more on spoken and written texts produced by the person with aphasia. This is in keeping with recent suggestions (evident also in this book) to focus on the social consequences of aphasia, using qualitative measures in concert with quantitative scoring and focus on conversation in intervention.

Do we need to address the power imbalance in the aphasia therapy interaction?

Unfortunately, it seems difficult to reverse the power imbalance in aphasia therapy interactions. Therapists cast themselves as experts who can influence communication problems. Typically they work in a medical or clinical setting. Even if therapy takes place in the community, perhaps in someone's home, the imbalance is always evident (Duchan *et al.* 1999). The client will always wait for the therapist to commence proceedings, to nominate topics, to be definite, to take over and to end the interaction. There is definitely a need to address this imbalance.

If the therapist only samples her client's communication in interactions with her in the session, access to the most important genre in that person's everyday life may be blocked. After all, the person with aphasia is attending therapy to improve their abilities at the conversational level. So the therapy should at least partly focus on this genre in some detail. Critical theorists point to the power that is inherent in language, that language defines the extent of our world, our access to developing social identity and our ability to access social life. Aphasia therapists are in the unique position of being able to empower clients to reacquire access to the various discourses they valued, such as the discourses associated with being a father, a friend, a social club member or a wife. It is therefore imperative that access be accorded to these genres by the therapists who essentially act as gatekeepers in this regard. It is unlikely that access to the restricted structured interview genre within a therapy room will have a significant effect on the person's ability to function across the range of discourses that were essential to them before their stroke. Without exposure to the conversations that were characteristic of the person's life, the therapist is denying that person the opportunity to work on the very skill they want to improve.

So what can be done to focus on conversation within the therapy setting?

Once there is a realization that the therapist's interaction with the person with aphasia may not be typical of other interactions, it is important to obtain a representative sample. One way of achieving this is by recording conversations on the telephone using an answering machine that enables two-way recording. A proviso with this is that both parties must be aware they are being recorded and provide prior consent in this regard. Such conversations can provide a wealth of information and insight into the power of context on language use. In a study of five people with traumatic brain injury (TBI) in interactions on the telephone with their mothers, therapists, the bus timetable information service and police officers, there were marked differences in language use by the people with TBI according to their communication partner. The five people with TBI were compared with their brothers across these interactions (Togher *et al.* 1997; Togher and Hand 1998). These differences were attributable to two main factors. First, the people with TBI were given different communicative opportunities according to who they spoke to. For example, the bus timetable service providers gave the people with TBI the opportunity to give information, ask questions and clarify information, whereas mothers tended to restrict the options of their sons with TBI by asking a limited set of questions to which they already knew the answer, failing to encourage elaboration on topics and making frequent requests for confirmation regarding accuracy of information. Therapist interactions were highly structured, with the typical initiation–response–feedback, a failure to encourage elaboration and use of interruptions, checking and confirmation requests when the person with TBI provided new information.

The second factor explaining differences across the four communication partners was the effect of the relationship between the participants and the effect of this on language use. The relationship between participants, also known as tenor, was varied in this study according to the variables of *status* (with the therapists and police officers having a professional status with some authority and power, mothers also having considerable status, authority and power and the bus timetable service providers have little authority or power); and *familiarity* (with mothers and therapists being more familiar than police or bus timetable service providers). These variations in tenor resulted in differences in language use. Interestingly, control subjects responded to a greater degree to the variation in tenor when compared with the people with TBI. In some cases the people with TBI did not respond to marked power imbalance. For example, some people with TBI used the police officer's first name, introduced unrelated topics and baldly asked for information with a failure to use politeness markers. While this has implications for TBI rehabilitation specifically, there are implications for people with aphasia from this research.

People with TBI are known to have difficulties accessing and responding to the interpersonal functions of language, such as being appropriately responsive to their communication partner, being aware of their contributions within the communicative process and having a concept of the overall structure of an interaction. In contrast, the interpersonal functions are usually quite intact for the person with aphasia and can therefore serve as strengths from which they can draw as they develop their modified social communicator self. Providing different communicative opportunities for the person allows for an expansion of the potential use of their linguistic resources, by providing communication partners who may provide more collaborative support (such as a familiar friend with a large amount of shared knowledge) during the interaction, or by providing genres which are less difficult because of increased structure (such as a simple face-to-face service encounter requiring less talk). In other words, therapy can be structured so that the person interacts with a range of people who vary according to power, status and authority.

Empowering the client can be done in a number of ways. Writing from a feminist discourse perspective, Poynton (1985) suggested that those in positions of power were more likely to be in information giving roles, would direct the interaction, nominate topics, and be more likely to interrupt and close the interaction. Extending these notions, one way of situating clients in more powerful positions is to place them in information giving roles where they have status and authority. This could include giving information to other people with aphasia, speaking to community groups, providing orientation to new clients or staff, or in other ways, handing over responsibility for information giving to the client. In a group setting, the chair of the group could be rotated on a weekly basis, so that all group members had the opportunity to nominate topics, be permitted to interrupt others and be responsible for closing discussion.

Another suggestion to facilitate the talk in the therapy session is by sharing an experience with the client so that you both have something to talk about later. The artificiality of the therapy context promotes the notion that all talk needs to be about activities that occur outside the therapy room and that have been undertaken by the client. Going shopping or to a museum, attending a cooking group or a mobility group, or even going with the client to the canteen for a cup of coffee can enable you both to share an experience together.

An example of sharing an experience arose for me when I was working with a 42-year-old woman who had global aphasia as a result of a left hemisphere haemorrhage. She could occasionally produce one or two words, but generally used a combination of gesture and drawing to get her message across. 'Conversation' in therapy was difficult, as she was only able to respond, and I had little information about her life prior to her stroke. This lady, Maria (not her real name), was a single mother with two school-age children, and lived in a house with a large back yard on the outskirts of Sydney. In collaboration with the social worker and occupational therapist, my brief was to assess whether she would be able to function independently if discharged home. We investigated whether Maria could plan a meal, go shopping for the ingredients, cook the dinner and interact with her children as they returned from school. The meal planning and shopping trip were quite successful, but on our return home we found, to our dismay, that the dog next door had killed the family's duck and left the remains in the back yard. As the children were about to arrive home from school, it became clear that we had to bury the duck quickly (which included picking up hundreds of feathers!) So the social worker and I commenced digging a hole in the vegetable patch, under the instruction of our client. At the time it was quite stressful, as Maria was upset about losing her duck and anxious lest the children see the mess in the back yard. Of course, later on we all had a laugh about it. It was after this incident that a real conversation occurred between Maria and myself. On our return to the unit, we jointly described our experience to some of the nursing staff. Maria's excellent use of gesture added to the clarity of the story, and there was a certain degree of solidarity as we had handled a crisis together. Our interactions after that time were different, with an increased ease of getting ideas across to each other. Clearly, our jointly constructed experience had helped us develop a shared history.

Ylvisaker (1998) describes the promotion of collaborative and elaborative talk as a strategy to assist people with traumatic brain injury to interact more effectively. The principle here is that people often produce joint narratives as they describe an experience they enjoyed together. Both participants are responsible for the collaboratively produced talk. Contrast the following examples:

Example 1

Therapist: *What did you do on Sunday?*
Client: *Bus . . . went over there.*
Therapist: *You went on a bus. Where did you go?*
Client: *Over there.*

Example 2

Therapist: *Wasn't that a great shopping trip?*
Client: *Yeah.*
Therapist: *What was that first place we went to with all those amazing cakes?*
Client: *Michel's . . . cakes . . . fattening.*
Therapist: *Oh one every now and then is OK – I'm sure chocolate must be good
              for you.*
Client: *And nice coffee too.*
Therapist: *Yes, we must go back there.*

In the first of these two examples, the therapist is in the role of demanding information, with no background or shared information. He does not provide information, give opinions or support the client in a collaborative manner. The second example shows the therapist jointly introducing the talking activity by appealing to recent shared knowledge. The client's conversation is supported by the therapist providing an opinion, giving positive comments related to the activity rather than critiquing the individual's grammar or lexis.

There are other ways of working with conversation within the therapy setting. The most obvious perhaps is, where possible, working with family members (for example, conversational coaching advocated by Holland 1991; Boles 1998; Wilkinson *et al.* 1998), training volunteers as advocated by the life participation movement (Lyon *et al.* 1997, Kagan *et al.* 2001; and others) and deriving therapy goals from a number of sources of discourse genres and communication partners who vary according to status and familiarity.

Aphasia therapists rarely observe the person with aphasia in interactions with their family, friends or in the community, usually as a result of time constraints, but also because they don't have a way of analysing these interactions. With the advent of e-therapy, video-phone link-ups and tele-health initiatives, it may be easier to observe the person with aphasia interacting with a range of communication partners without their presence being required in the therapy room. Similarly, as therapists become more familiar with sociolinguistic methods of analysis they may be more likely to look beyond the therapy room and their own interactions for insight into how a person with aphasia really converses.

So, what are the implications of all this? Acknowledging the fact that we have interviews and not conversations in therapy may be a big leap for some. It implies that we need to find out how the person *really* converses with people in *their* world. Being aware that traditional assessment scores may provide little insight into the mechanisms of communication is another conceptual step. This implies that we need to seek out other ways of evaluating the texts that are produced in the therapy context. This doesn't discount the value of the therapy interaction – there is much to be learned from how a person communicates with a therapist. However, the therapy interaction does not represent how that person will function in other contexts. Much more can be learned from other sources, such as recording real conversations with other people who vary according to familiarity and power, and from evaluating these using sociolinguistic methods.

Becoming aware of the power imbalance that exists in therapy interactions can be a revelation in itself. In my own case, I am now increasingly aware of how the therapy interaction can be modified by shifting the power imbalance ever so slightly. So, rather than simply asking questions in an interview format (and therefore being a requester), I am now more likely to give information to the client regarding my own personal experience. For example, if we are talking about places to go at the weekend, I'll contribute with places I have been to recently and recount the sequence of events, as well as giving an opinion. This harks back to the basis of PACE therapy (Davis and Wilcox 1985) where the therapist takes turns in guessing and giving information. I am suggesting something more, however, as the therapist is giving something of their identity, their self, rather than simply describing a picture. Once you've given some information, it doesn't take the client long to feel the shift in the usual power structure and start asking occasional questions. This is where something approximating 'conversation' can happen. The amount and type of information I would divulge to a client obviously varies from client to client. Some clients clearly prefer the therapist to determine the course of events and feel uncomfortable with asking questions in a conversational manner. In these cases other strategies need to be put in place to foster conversation. Sometimes a more collaborative relationship can develop. In other words, facilitating a shift in power can have profound implications for promoting conversation.

If a therapist has these ideas in mind, the person with aphasia is more likely to receive a fair and appropriate service, respond to therapy positively and engage in a more collaborative and shared experience with the therapist. Ideally these approaches lead to a greater involvement of others in the therapy process, including friends, family and even local shopkeepers, with the outcome being improved jointly constructed texts, and the continuing development of both a shared and a new personal identity.

References

Armstrong, E. (1992) Clause complex relations in aphasic discourse: a longitudinal case study, *Journal of Neurolinguistics*, 7(4): 261–75.

Armstrong, E. (2000) Aphasic discourse analysis: the story so far, *Aphasiology*, 14(9): 875–92.

Boles, L. (1998) Conversational discourse analysis as a method for evaluating progress in aphasia: a case report, *Journal of Communication Disorders*, 31: 261–74.

Davis, G. and Wilcox, J. (1985) *Adult Aphasia Rehabilitation: Applied Pragmatics*. San Diego; CA: College-Hill Press.

Duchan, J., Maxwell, M. and Kovarsky, D. (1999) Evaluating competence in the course of everyday interaction, in D. Kovarsky, J. Duchan and M. Maxwell (eds) *Constructing (In)competence: Disabling Evaluations in Clinical and Social Interactions*. London: Erlbaum.

Ferguson, A. (1994) The influence of aphasia, familiarity and activity on repair, *Aphasiology*, 8: 143–57.

Halliday, M.A.K. (1994) *An Introduction to Functional Grammar* (2nd edn). London: Edward Arnold.

Holland, A.L. (1991) Pragmatic aspects of intervention in aphasia, *Journal of Neurolinguistics*, 6(2): 197–211.

Holmes, J. (1992) *An Introduction to Sociolinguistics*. London: Longman.

Kagan, A., Black, S., Duchan, J., Simmons-Mackie, N. and Square, P. (2001) Training volunteers as conversational partners using 'Supported Conversation with Adults with Aphasia' (SCA): a controlled trial, *Journal of Speech, Language and Hearing Research*, 44: 624–38.

Kovarsky, D., Kimbarow, M. and Kastner, D. (1999) The construction of incompetence during group therapy with traumatically brain injured adults, in D. Kovarsky, J. Duchan and M. Maxwell (eds) *Constructing (In)competence: Disabling Evaluations in Clinical and Social Interactions*. London: Erlbaum.

Lyon, J., Cariski, D., Keisler, L. *et al.* (1997) Communication partners: enhancing participation in life and communication for adults with aphasia in natural settings, *Aphasiology*, 11: 693–708.

Modjeska, D. (1999) *Stravinksy's Lunch*. Sydney: Picador.

Parr, S. (1996) Everyday literacy in aphasia: radical approaches to functional assessment and therapy, *Aphasiology*, 10(5): 469–503.

Poynton, C. (1985) *Language and Gender: Making the Difference*. Victoria: Deakin University Press.

Silvast, M. (1991) Aphasia therapy dialogues, *Aphasiology*, 5: 383–90.

Simmons-Mackie, N. (2000) Social approaches to the management of aphasia, in L. Worrall and C. Frattali (eds) *Neurogenic Communication Disorders: A Functional Approach*. New York: Thieme.

Togher, L., Hand, L. and Code, C. (1997) Analysing discourse in the traumatic brain injury population: telephone interactions with different communication partners, *Brain Injury*, 11(3): 169–89.

Togher, L. and Hand, L. (1998) Use of politeness markers with different communication partners: an investigation of five subjects with traumatic brain injury, *Aphasiology*, 12(7/8): 491–504.

Togher, L. (2001) Discourse sampling in the 21st century, *Journal of Communication Disorders*, 34(1/2): 131–50.

Wilkinson, R., Bryan, K., Lock, S. *et al.* (1998) Therapy using conversation analysis: helping couples adapt to aphasia in conversation, *International Journal of Language and Communication Disorders*, 33(Suppl.): 144–9.

Ylvisaker, M. (1998) *Traumatic Brain Injury Rehabilitation: Children and Adolescents.* Boston, MA: Butterworth-Heinemann.

Acknowledgement

Many thanks to Dr Elizabeth Armstrong for her comments on this chapter.

8

Doing less, being more

Harry Clarke

Key points

- Harry Clarke is a counsellor and a person who has aphasia.
- In this chapter he talks about his philosophy of doing counselling and tells the story of his stroke and how he became a counsellor.
- Harry talks about the conditions and techniques which help the counselling process:
  - being a good listener;
  - listening beyond words;
  - using the silences to focus on the client and their feelings;
  - developing trust;
  - building a relationship with the person who comes to counselling.
- Harry encourages clients with aphasia to communicate in different ways.
- He talks about the different stages of grieving and gives some examples from his own experience.
- For Harry it is important to learn to 'just be' with a client, to focus totally on them – not to feel you have to do things and say things.

If I keep from meddling with people, they take care of themselves,
If I keep from commanding people, they behave themselves,
If I keep from preaching at people, they improve themselves,
If I keep from imposing on people, they become themselves.

(Lao Tse, quoted in Rogers 1980: 42)

I first read this saying by Lao Tse in Carl Rogers's book, *A Way of Being*. Lao Tse was a Zen Buddhist and Chinese sage who lived some 25 centuries ago. Rogers (the founder of person-centred psychotherapy and counselling) admits this saying is an oversimplification but, like him, I find it is one which resonates deeply with me. I guess the principle that less is more is not a new one. This forms part of my philosophy on counselling. It looks like a simple and uncomplicated philosophy but very often it is the simple things that need the most work. Later in this chapter I shall attempt to capture a flavour of this personal approach to counselling in describing how I worked with and learnt from a particular client who came for counselling.

Every client I see will have differing and changing needs as they move through a process of grieving. Often, this demands from me a more proactive input, especially in later stages of this process where the emphasis is more likely to be on a client's personal aims or goals. Part of this chapter therefore will look at some of my own journey through the grieving process and my own changing needs. Whether I am just being with a client early on, or offering a more practical view later on, I believe that the art of listening to another person is a real gift that is of immeasurable value to the healing process.

At this point, I make no excuse for quoting a passage from Rogers's chapter on experiences of communication. I use this extract to help illustrate the conditions I strive to provide with and for clients and that contribute greatly to any therapeutic relationship:

A creative, active, sensitive, accurate, empathic, nonjudgmental listening is for me terribly important in a relationship. It is important for me to provide it; it has been extremely important, especially at certain times in my life, to receive it. I feel that I have grown within myself when I have provided it; I am very sure that I have grown and been released and enhanced when I have received this kind of listening
(Rogers 1980: 14)

One of the many important benefits, I believe, of listening at the deep level Rogers describes is that it allows clients to feel valued especially when they may be experiencing feelings of vulnerability due to loss. Listening at this deep level can sometimes go beyond the mere use of words for it can allow for an existential closeness that helps do away with the need to intellectualize. I believe that it is within this closeness that you really do begin to hear another person. Carl Rogers continues to be the biggest influence on my counselling work.

My own process towards becoming a counsellor began, unbeknown to me, one day late in June 1988. Upon awakening one particular morning I became immediately aware that things were wrong. My right side was heavy and numb. Struggling to the phone and calling a friend only brought more fearful confusion. As I tried to tell him my problem I realized I was not making sense. I was not talking. Time and again I tried, but no words would come, not even my own name, just this jumbled panicky noise. An ambulance was alerted and soon I found myself beginning day one of a three-month stay in hospital where eventually I would begin the long road back to recovery by having speech, physio- and occupational therapies. In the early days of this recovery I had quickly moved from initial shock in the form of closing down, into a strong denial of the consultant's diagnosis of stroke.

It must have been around six weeks into this stay in hospital, while I was receiving therapies for the physical problems left by the stroke, that I began to move out of denial. Denial had done its job by shielding me from the enormity of my illness, and was now slowly being replaced by an angry and distressing reality. The emotional fallout left by the stroke, the thoughts and the feelings I was experiencing were starting to spill over as a sense of desperation began to take hold. I yearned for somewhere or someone to bring these intensely uncomfortable feelings to. It seemed that any help was confined to purely physical difficulties. Emotions on the other hand, were, it seemed, my business and I would have to deal with them by myself. Regrettably, I was forced to take extreme measures. I knew speech therapy was important, but these feelings had taken precedence over everything else. It is said action speaks louder than words so by sweeping everything off the therapist's desk I was expressing the desperation I felt. I have spoken and written of this dramatic event many times (Clarke 1998). Indeed it was the first of several significant moments where I believe seeds were sown that would eventual grow towards my becoming a counsellor.

Until my stay in hospital I had, in my ignorance, not heard of speech therapy. Indeed, it took a few sessions with the therapist before I could fully appreciate what she was doing. She was helping me to communicate; she was helping me to talk. She very quickly became vitally important to me; I liked and trusted her. I also admired her for the work she had chosen to do. I remember thinking, 'What a wonderfully worthwhile and helpful thing to do'. I also imagined how rewarding this kind of work might be. It was, though, the quality of the relationship between myself and the speech therapist that I was to learn from. A quality that was just not present with other therapists. This was greatly enhanced by these sessions being on a one-to-one basis. It would be gratifying to hear her door close and know the focus for the hour was on improving my communication. I had quickly realized that my time with her was all-important. It was not surprising then that it was to her I brought all my fears.

I clearly recall the therapist looking somewhat alarmed as the contents of her desk hit the floor, as I poured out my confused and angry feelings. But this demonstration of emotion needed her presence. I needed her acknowledgement of my predicament and she gave me this by giving me the time and the space to express myself. When later I asked myself what she had done, the answer I arrived at was 'not that much', or at least that's how it appeared. I cannot recall her saying one single word. What she silently gave me though was precious time and space. Granted I had initially to push for this, but when we realized that my need was greater than hers, her agenda was put on hold. I recall leaving that therapy room at the end of the session feeling a real sense of relief. It had been, in essence, a purely cathartic release.

I do not know if this therapist had counselling training, but allowing me to try to express these feelings was the best and most helpful thing anyone could do for me at that point. This was an early example of doing less that I have learnt from. I have, through this and other experiences, become more comfortable in the presence of painful emotions, allowing clients to express them in whatever way they need to. What helps me here is knowing that to soothe or calm a client is often to do them a disservice. It can be an intrusion into their grieving. Just being with them and conveying a warmth, understanding and acceptance will provide a client with the right conditions to begin to tap into their own innate self-healing processes. For me the reward is that my presence will have played a part.

Perhaps the best example I can give where I used this past experience in my own work was while working with Ellen, a woman who had had a stroke just two years after her husband of 35 years had died. At our introductory session we spent some time together and I explained how the service might be of help to her. Ellen was easy to like. My first impressions were of someone low in confidence and somewhat withdrawn. The stroke had left her with no intelligible words and right-sided weakness. Ellen had still been grieving for her husband when her illness struck, compounding that grief and adding to its intensity. Ellen was, not surprisingly, experiencing a deep sense of loss. The first step was to begin to build a relationship between us through trust. We did this at a steady and comfortable pace. I would remind her that each session would last for one hour, adding that there was no set limit to the amount of sessions and that we would review our work periodically. Early sessions were spent getting to know each other better and finding Ellen's preferred methods of communication. These were using her personal communication book, writing (in the form of one or two words) and the occasional, and generally accurate, 'Yes' or 'No'. Ellen used body language and facial expressions to great effect. This helped with communication by backing up and verifying anything she had written during a session.

As Ellen became more relaxed and comfortable during sessions she began writing significant names and dates. These included close family members, in particular her husband, and dates of importance. I explored the significance of every date with her: birthdays and anniversaries, the date of her stroke and that of her husband's death. Often she would tearfully return to this last date. At these times, I would endeavour to get close to what it was Ellen was experiencing. I would be quiet and still. I would concentrate on my presence and focus my full attention on Ellen. It was not so important to know exactly what it was that Ellen was communicating. That could come later if she wished. The important thing at these moments was just being with her in as non-intrusive a way as I could. One such session took place on an important anniversary of her wedding and Ellen was particularly upset as she wrote first her name then her husband's followed by the date of her wedding. I said no more than a handful of words throughout the hour long session, during which time Ellen, between tears, would write other significant dates, peoples' ages and countries she and her husband had visited together. Mostly though, she cried. As the session came toward its end Ellen glanced at the clock and then began to write first my name, under which she wrote 'thank you' and beneath that she wrote her name in full. Then, with some difficulty, she stood up and in silence collected her things and left.

It's hard to do justice to this encounter in the written word except to say that at times during this session there was felt to be a healing presence between us. Now, I know that this may sound fanciful, but there was indeed a powerful positive presence within the counselling room that was almost tangible. As I sat alone for some time afterwards reflecting and making notes on this I became aware of feeling quietly privileged and somewhat humbled by the experience. It may all sound a bit heavy, but I assure you, as sessions developed, Ellen the person began to re-emerge. She became more expressive, smiled (indeed laughed) often, and in certain sessions Ellen would even sing significant songs. These songs were recognizable only by their tune but they were produced with gusto and emotion.

Over a few months, Ellen's whole demeanour had changed. She had become more alive and self-confident. How had I helped? First, I began to listen and to tune into where she was emotionally. By offering Ellen the three core conditions of empathy, genuineness and non-possessive warmth, we very quickly built trust between us. These core conditions formed a growth-inducing climate. Importantly, in this climate I believe Ellen could not help but feel valued, enabling her self-esteem, self-worth and confidence to grow. This was in turn reinforced by the whole enabling culture of Connect, the centre in which I work. Second, I listened to myself and monitored my own feelings throughout the sessions. This is important because to join with a client and offer a high degree of empathetic understanding leaves a risk of emotional over-involvement.

Many years ago, I remember reading that emotions can be likened to viruses, in that they can be infectious and easy to catch. Staying with this analogy, how do I keep myself from dis-ease when exposed to a client's emotional pain? As soon as I begin to experience a client's pain excessively I set about grounding myself. For me, being grounded means being calm, centred, focused and ready to be of use. First, I relax my body (which, as a sign to me, will have tensed up) by regulating my breathing. Then I move back emotionally for a while. This will allow me to connect more fully with my client.

Being grounded helps me to manage difficult moments in counselling and this was particularly the case when I first started working as a counsellor. An early difficulty was, ironically, dealing with silences and my need sometimes to fill them. I knew that the client's needs were paramount and that my discomfort with silences would put me in danger of doing them a disservice. So, by reflecting on the nature of silences in the counselling process and exploring these in supervision sessions, I gained a fresh perspective on them and their usefulness. After all, to process thoughts and feelings, some of which can be complex or painful, can take time. To take a client away from this quiet process before they have been able fully to engage with it would, in effect, be my difficulty and would be a failing on my part. There will always be a small part of me that will desire or wish to fix things, to make things better for us both. I guess that this is second nature when faced with emotional distress, but by awareness and becoming more comfortable in the presence of another's pain it becomes easier to resist what would in effect be my own issue, leaving me again more able just to be with the client.

As stated earlier most, if not all, the clients I see will be grieving for their loss and will be at a different stage of the grieving process when they come to counselling. These stages will be determined by several factors ranging from the time since the onset of aphasia, its severity, the family support network available, the client's character and any other disabilities. Having an adequate understanding of these stages and recognizing where a client might be in this process is important as this will help me to tune in and understand more clearly where they might be coming from.

This feels like a good point to mention Elizabeth Kubler Ross, who was one of the first people to describe the stages of the grieving process. During my training I first became aware of her groundbreaking book, *On Death and Dying* (1969). I still remember feeling mixed emotions as our course tutors led a discussion on her, her work and the stages of the grieving process. To be able to explore, name and give a likely sequence to these different stages was a revelation to me as I already knew these stages intimately. OK, emotions such as anger and depression (and even denial) were quite easy for me to spot, but bargaining, resolution, personal growth – these were new terms that helped me understand at a deeper level my own grieving process, and even the fact that I was still in it!

According to Kubler Ross, the most important stages and their usual sequence are:

- Shock
- Denial
- Anger
- Depression
- Bargaining
- Realism
- Acceptance/Resolution
- Readjustment
- Personal growth

Seeing those stages neatly listed of course belies the complexity of this process and will offer only a guide as to what a client experiencing loss may be feeling at any given time. It is very likely, however, that a sudden and catastrophic event such as stroke and aphasia may engender strong and intense feelings of loss, as was the case with me.

Some of the stages above are quite familiar, but others less so. To give an example of bargaining, which is one of the least talked about stages, I thought I would use my own personal experience as an illustration. For me bargaining had more far reaching consequences than I could ever have imagined.

The stage (or phase) of bargaining is one that people will often go through without others knowing, and so it was for me. During my three month stay in hospital, one routine among many was finding myself being wheeled into the physiotherapy department and placed beside a large notice board while I waited until the therapist was ready for me. During these periods I would look at and try to read the many posters and notices that had been placed there, even though in those early days and weeks (much to my distress) they made little or no sense to me. As the weeks turned into months, I was slowly beginning to understand some of the smaller words and would focus on one large poster in particular to gauge my progress. Then the day arrived when I could, with some difficulty, read and understand sufficiently all the words that were on it. This alone would be cause for celebration, but it was what was written on the poster that still resonates with me today.

The poster was by the Stroke Association and asked for volunteers to visit people recovering from stroke in the hospital for one or two hours a week. Now, I would not say I was a particularly religious person but at that moment I found myself entering into a deal with God. I promised at that moment to visit people with strokes if I could, in return, walk and talk again. I would reinforce this pledge every time I saw the poster, right up until leaving hospital and moving to a rehabilitation centre in Wimbledon.

At the rehabilitation centre, I was beginning to feel better about my recovery. I felt as if my old self was slowly returning: I was coming back.

This optimistic view was being helped enormously by the obvious improvements in my speech and articulation. Earlier feelings of vulnerability were slowly dissipating. I was feeling stronger, not just physically but emotionally, so much so that I felt I was able and willing to listen to others and their stories, some of which were distressing. Very often, the only thing I could do was listen (something I mistakenly thought was inadequate). I berated the lack of trained help in the area of rehabilitation counselling. I was slowly beginning to identify an unmet need and more seeds were being sown.

There were, of course, certain patients and their situations that I found upsetting, maybe more so because I was still in the grieving process myself. My own emotions were still pretty raw and I found that I was sensitive to others. One particular patient, indeed the very first patient I had met at the centre, had had a severe stroke which had affected both her left and right side as well as impairing her speech. I admired her courage and I was inspired by her often cheerful, always optimistic outlook to what was obviously going to be a long and unenviable journey of recovery.

By contrast one journey we did all enjoy was the one home for the weekend. As we waited in the communal recreational room for our various modes of transport to arrive I heard her begin to cry, a painfully distressing crying that seemed to be coming from somewhere deep inside. I guessed that something had gone wrong with her weekend plans. I was concerned as to what could be wrong, what was causing her so much sorrow. I asked the nurse why she was so upset and I was reluctantly told that her partner was at the last moment unable to pick her up to attend her young daughters' birthday celebrations. The nurse then added that it was exactly a year to the day, at the previous birthday party, that she had had the stroke. This irony seemed particularly cruel and left me with such a feeling of helplessness as to make me wonder what anyone could do for her.

There were other such moments in my three-month stay at the centre that I can still recall vividly even 12 years later. This, I believe, is testimony to the powerful effect other patients and their struggles were having on me. I had entered into another way of being, that of a person with an acquired disability. My goal, though, was complete recovery and at the time this goal still felt achievable for me. But for some . . . I would wonder. I would often catch myself feeling for others then quickly remind myself that I wasn't quite out of the woods yet myself. I was, however, without forethought, developing a greater capacity to care; to care for others whose predicaments often seemed, to my untrained eye, almost hopeless. Despite this, I rarely sensed defeat in others at the centre and this on occasions was an uplifting experience. It is said that a person's true character is often shown in adversity when you are forced to call on resources and qualities you may not have been aware of possessing. I saw plenty of examples of this, not least my own, at the rehabilitation centre.

I was discharged from the centre as it closed shortly before the Christmas break. For me, though, the reality was that I still had a lot of work ahead to achieve my 'complete recovery'. At the beginning of 1989 I returned to hospital, only this time of my own volition. I had asked if I could use the physiotherapy department resources and spent many mornings that year working on improving the function of my right arm and leg. These mornings also began to serve my reluctant yet steadily growing acceptance that a full recovery may well be beyond me. I would play a recurring scenario in my head where I would be at a social function of some kind and would be asked by a stranger within minutes of meeting them what I did for a living. I would shudder at the only response I could honestly give, 'Well er nothing because . . .' If I did not want this fantasy to become a reality I would have someway, somehow, to reinvent myself.

But as what? My options appeared to be few. On reflection, I realize that I was between the stages of acceptance and readjustment and I stayed in this limbo until early 1990. At this point, my view of the future was given voice in a period I shall call the 'moaning stage', as this is what I seemed to do most, especially in the presence of the therapists at the hospital.

It was during this moaning phase that a therapist, tired of my oft repeated assertion about lack of counselling support, stopped me in my tracks and said rather curtly, 'Instead of moaning why not do a counselling course? You do it!' Importantly, she added that she thought I might make a good counsellor and she agreed that there was a real need for this service.

This suggestion, coupled with a broken romance, led to an initially desperate embracing of spiritual healing. Then ever so slowly the surprisingly simple and obvious answer became clear. It's there right in front of you! A different poster . . . same message . . . remember . . . the deal. I pondered for many days and weeks whether this was the way to go, and what of my declaration? If I were to make a promise then break a promise it would be highly unwise to choose such an omnipresent recipient to renege against . . . I mean, let's face it, He would be sure to know.

The time had come for personal growth.The seeds that had been planted during my physical rehabilitation now needed careful nurturing. I had found my direction and I could at last begin my long sought-for reinvention: that of becoming a trained counsellor.

Personal growth, the longest and in many respects the most important stage in the grieving process also encompasses the final stage of growth: that of death itself. Therefore it is the one stage where being stuck in it is to be actively encouraged. For me personally this importantly on-going stage has helped me to reflect on my own experiences and, in turn, has shaped my counselling style which is underpinned by the 'doing less, being more' philosophy. The beginning of this stage can, as with me, be an exciting and challenging time for clients. It can also be sweetly liberating and will often require from me a more proactive role. This is combined, as always, with a process of listening carefully and looking out for a client's vagaries, inferences and half-formed ideas (even those thoughts which may be on the periphery of awareness), striving to accurately track them by reflecting back what I hear, and on some occasions even that which I do not hear. I will have changed my stance, becoming more flexible, and may challenge or reframe these thoughts or ideas if it feels helpful. I can do this because, having built and established trust in the relationship, I will have allowed myself now to do that bit more in the form of trusting my own and my client's intuitive responses. I am aware that in this healthy and positive climate a client will have already begun to work toward tapping into their own self-actualizing tendencies, in their own search for a worthwhile and rewarding disabled identity. My overall role in this process is one of having been but a brief companion.

Doing less and being more has helped me as a counsellor and in other areas of my life where quality listening is called for. Anyone can begin to improve the quality of their listening by first slowing the pace down, as this will help in being more grounded. While putting your own agenda aside, try to focus 100 per cent on the person you are communicating with. Do not offer advice, and resist looking for a place to jump in. Concentrate instead on understanding the other person and connecting with them. If and when you feel you want to say something, wait, don't speak for two or three seconds or stay quiet for as long as is comfortable. These silent moments really can be golden and will often be the most revealing for the person you have heard and you in turn will be offering help that is genuinely helpful.

I opened this chapter with some thoughts I had found from Lao Tse taken from Carl Rogers's book, *A Way Of Being*. I would like to close in the same way, for I believe that the following passages capture the essence of the doing less being more philosophy that I try to adhere to as a counsellor:

A leader is best
When people barely know that he exists
Not so good when people obey and acclaim him,
Worst when they despise him . . .
But of a good leader, who talks little,
When his work is done, his aim fulfilled,
They will all say, 'We did this ourselves'.
It is as though he listened,

And such listening as his enfolds us in a silence
In which at last we begin to hear
What we are meant to be.
　　　　　(Lao Tse, cited in Rogers 1980: 42)

References

Kubler Ross, E. (1969) *On Death and Dying*. New York: Scribner.
Clarke, H. (1998) Harry's story: becoming a counsellor following a stroke, in D. Syder (ed.) *Wanting to Talk: Case Studies in Communication Disorders*. London: Whurr Publishers.
Rogers, C. (1980) *A Way of Being*. Boston: Houghton Mifflin.

9

Changing places: reflections of
therapists and group members on
the power and potential of groups

Tom Penman and Turid de Mare

Key points

- Tom and Turid are both therapists – Turid worked as a psychotherapist and Tom works as a speech and language therapist. Turid
  has aphasia and Tom works in a centre for people with aphasia.
- In this chapter they talk about their experiences of working with
  groups – as therapists and as group members.
- In the beginning Tom found working with people in groups very
  challenging – he didn't know what to do or how to deal with the
  real life issues that people in the group wanted to talk about.
- Turid says different groups have different agendas and groups
  change over time.
- She feels the important thing about groups is being together and
  thinking together.
- Everyone in the group has a responsibility to make it work – not
  just the group facilitator.
- Turid and Tom talk about how therapists can find it difficult to
  give up power and control but in groups it's important that the
  therapist isn't the 'boss'.
- They say group facilitators need to learn to believe in the skills and
  expertise of group members.
- They think its very important for facilitators to reflect on the way
  they work in groups but a lot of therapists don't get much training
  and support for working with groups.

Introduction

Group therapy with people with aphasia has a long tradition, but has remained in the background of much clinical practice and research (Elman 1999). Research studies have mainly concentrated on the features and efficacy of particular group interventions. Furthermore, speech and language therapy education in working with groups has predominantly focused on skill-building and working to specific communicative outcomes. Within clinical education and practice there has been less of a focus on the process and dynamics of group work.

This chapter looks explicitly at the experience and process of group therapy. It is based on a series of in-depth interviews between Turid, a group psychotherapist who has acquired aphasia following a stroke, and Tom, a speech and language therapist working with people with aphasia. The process of writing for the two of us has been an interesting and evolving one. Taped conversations between us were followed up by written summaries of the key themes. This led to further discussion and amendment of those points. Tom wrote up the bulk of the chapter, with Turid reviewing and editing the drafts. This final version is a mix of our individual and combined voices including our personal stories and quotes from our taped discussions.

We have both been participants in, and facilitators of, groups. In this chapter we draw on our insider perspectives of group processes in aphasia therapy and psychotherapy to highlight issues related to the focus, direction and planning of aphasia groups. We explore the themes of what group therapy is and can be, and why groups work effectively. Drawing parallels with group psychotherapy practice and training, we discuss the importance of attention to group process and dynamics in creating conditions for authentic learning and change in everyday life for those with aphasia.

Tom's story

I trained as a speech and language therapist. Initially I worked with children and adults with a wide variety of communication disabilities, across a number of settings – including health centres, schools, hospitals, day centres and in people's homes. Although most of my work was done on a one-to-one basis (and often behind closed doors or curtains) I also worked with groups, most of which had begun with a different therapist. These groups included aphasia groups, children's language groups, laryngectomee support groups and reminiscence groups with people with dementia.

I found many of these groups daunting and exhausting. This was particularly true for the groups of people with aphasia which had been running for a number of years before my involvement. I had had no specific training in how to facilitate groups and was personally unclear about the benefits of group work over individual treatment. I was a young and newly qualified therapist still unsure of my skills and authority, so entering a room with up to 12 people with varying and sometimes complex needs filled me with fear and trepidation. Groups, however, appeared to be a convenient way of treating more people within a given time, thereby reducing the waiting list.

Lacking a clear long-term rationale for aphasia group work, I tended to focus on specific communication tasks and activities for each session. I chose these tasks to match the specific skills that I perceived important to build for group members, for example, word finding or gesture. This was also often in the context of a wide mix of skills, needs and abilities within the groups. Issues that arose, such as feelings and emotions or dealing with finance and benefits, I often viewed as outside my remit as a speech and language therapist. I would briefly acknowledge the personal comments but then either move back quickly to the communication task at hand, or else 'subvert' the comments into communication activities, for example, generating synonyms of words to do with feelings! In the end, my discomfort and dissatisfaction persisted. I perceived the open-ended aphasia groups as having a limited ability to impact on the participants' linguistic processing, which I then felt was my job. I didn't know how to move people on, so I discharged them. Group participants' reactions to being discharged was strong and negative, but at the time I felt 'professionally' justified and stood my ground.

The other groups I was involved in seemed to me to have a clearer focus and rationale. The laryngectomee group was set up to pass on information and practical skills. The format included presentations from members of the Ear, Nose and Throat (ENT) team followed by short question and answer sessions. Although there was space for sharing of experiences and group bonding, I saw these as peripheral to the important educational role of the group. The children's language groups again followed an apparently clear agenda. They resulted from extensive assessment of the childrens' receptive and expressive language skills, and were made up of activities that aimed to train language concepts tested in language batteries. After the intervention period, the children, unsurprisingly, tended to show improvements on the same language batteries that were used in the assessment. Interestingly, and somewhat worryingly in retrospect, we did not always think to find out what impact these assessment changes might or might not have had on the childrens' communication and interactions at home or at school, or on their self-perceptions and well-being.

Soon after disbanding the open-ended aphasia groups, I joined a psychotherapy training course run by the local psychology department. I felt I needed more information and techniques to cope with the emotional issues that were 'seeping out' from clients during my therapy sessions. Part of the training involved becoming a participant in a group myself, much to my surprise and anxiety! The style of the psychotherapist 'facilitating' the group was very different to my more didactic approach. She most often sat back and said nothing. There were long silences and eruptions of anger and frustration from group members at not being guided in what to talk about and do. It took a long time to develop any sense of trust between group members, but issues raised began to funda-mentally challenge the way I perceived the world and how I reacted to people. It was powerful and sometimes scary stuff. It was this experience that began to reveal to me something of what people with a communica-tion disability might feel on joining a group. It was also very different in feel and content to the groups I had run. I was not given answers but, rather, was encouraged to reflect on my motivations, assumptions and behaviours. I started to think about how people change and learn – maybe there were different ways to the 'therapist as expert' model I carried with me.

My style of working with groups has changed over the years, particu-larly as my philosophy of what therapy is about has evolved. Working with groups of people with aphasia at Connect has allowed me to see the wider context in which therapy can operate. In this work I have been strongly influenced by disability studies writers and my colleagues at Connect (Swain *et al.* 1993; Byng *et al.* 2000; Pound *et al.* 2000). Com-munication does not happen in a vacuum. Neither do stroke and aphasia. Life, relationships and the sense of who you are as a person in your community are affected. Therapy must, I feel, reflect these profound life changes, and group therapy is a great way of sharing complexities. Striving to work in a less didactic way has made me acknowledge more explicitly the expertise and skills of the group participants (which often they themselves may not readily recognize or acknowledge). It has also meant being prepared to be more responsive to the diverse issues that people with aphasia and their families and friends bring with them to the group through their experience of living with a communication disability. It is not so easy to contain and control what I might have once seen as 'messy' issues when I am trying to take the focus off myself as sole 'expert'. Instead I aim to foster conditions in which a group can start to take on the issues themselves. Taking risks, albeit calculated, has become more of a daily part of my practice. Having time and space to air these uncertainties and challenges, for example, through dedicated one-to-one supervision, team meetings and open discussion with group participants, have been crucial in supporting me at Connect to develop this different way of working.

Turid's story

I came over to England from Norway in my early twenties and married over here. My husband was a psychiatrist and psychotherapist. I was working in interior design when I first became interested in training as a psychotherapeutic counsellor myself. In the beginning, however, I didn't want to think about psychoanalysis, because it sounds so crazy!

I went to a group in my thirties because I wanted to know what happened in groups. I was very frightened of other people. For me, at the start, I thought they all talked much better than I could, as I wasn't English. Then as the group went on, people who had been very difficult changed. The people who came were doctors, nurses and psychotherapists, or just ordinary people who were interested in groups.

I went on to attend the introductory course of the Group Analytic Society. I was strongly influenced by the work of Foulkes, who developed small group work from Northfield Military hospital during World War Two (Foulkes and Anthony 1957). Then I got a job at MIND, the mental health charity, where I worked with groups of people with schizophrenia and depression. I was quite good at helping people to not have rows and finding out why people were so miserable and what might help. Some people came because their doctor had suggested the group, and others because they wanted to have therapy, but also to see and meet other people.

In 1999 I had a stroke. When I first got ill, I couldn't talk. I used to see one speech therapist, but felt sort of bereft, like there wasn't anybody else who talked like me. So I saw this person for an hour once a week. I tried to write. The person who came was very strident. She said to Pat, my husband, and me there were certain things we should do like Scrabble, and Pat absolutely hates Scrabble! And I was supposed to do it. It never worked! So then I saw an Australian lady and she was very nice.

Turid: *It was very funny because she tried to talk . . . Scribble . . . no . . . The tiny little . . . rushing around . . . scribble . . . it's an animal . . . a squirrel . . .*
Tom: *So you had to practice saying the word 'squirrel'?*
Turid: *Yes . . . I still can't do it!*

She said I would never be able to speak like before, and I thought that was such a downing thing to say, and I thought, 'ugh!'

I came along to Connect last year. I have been a part of various groups, each of which has felt different. Some have worked for me, others not so much. I feel that early on at Connect I talked about lots of practical issues in dealing with communication problems in my life. More recently I have joined a conversation group which takes a different focus. We have a simple sort of agenda where we think of a topic the week before to discuss. Some people bring pictures and drawings the following week and we talk. Sometimes we have to wait until somebody either has to say it again or say it several times, but it's like trying to create something. For me, that's the thing about groups – that you are able to communicate and be creative.

I went to a different group on a Friday morning. It was initially a place where we just talked about what we wanted rather than suddenly having an agenda. We started with one topic and then went on to talk about whatever else was going on. Often people would describe interests or parts of their lives that would not have emerged if there had been a tight agenda. We just hung out together! However, I was away for a while and when I came back there was a very definite agenda, about using the telephone. It felt different – it didn't feel so creative.

For me, as a member of groups of people with aphasia, the important thing is that when we talk everybody's mind is trying to reflect on what we have been thinking and what we are trying to say. Although it takes some time with aphasia, you can still think. In general, however, it's very easy not to think, even if you don't have aphasia!

Aphasia therapy and psychotherapy: comparisons and contentions

Through discussion of our experience of groups, we arrived at certain themes we felt show the similarities and differences between aphasia therapy and psychotherapy in groups. These themes relate particularly to participation and facilitation.

Being a group participant

Both of us had experienced belonging to psychotherapy groups. Conflict and the relationship with the group facilitator were common themes. We had both felt a good deal of anxiety and pressure on first joining our groups, not quite knowing what to expect and how to interact. Strong emotions and personal insecurity emerged for us both quite early on in the life of the groups. This resulted in the expectation that the therapist would come in and sort out the 'problem'. In neither of our experiences did the therapist take on this role. This caused us and some of the other members of our groups (those who remained!) to begin to reflect on our own motivations and assumptions, and perhaps begin to realize that our own world view wasn't the only one!

Anyway, it was all difficult . . . first people tried to say 'What's happening with me? How awful I was', then they changed and it was quite interesting to find how people, you know, they have little ideas and when they have to relate back, when they get on 'What was that about? Why did that happen?' . . . Then of course when it went on, people realized it was nothing to do with me, but them. And that was quite interesting, you know, that it's not they: 'I was absolutely wonderful', but they realized what happens with themselves and that was really what the . . . what was happening . . . you know, how often you of other people and don't think about yourself.

Turid

We reflected on the changes in group participation caused by aphasia. We tried to unpick what might be a direct result of the aphasia, and what was a normal part of group process. One issue that seemed to be a mix of the two was the difficulty at times of thinking and reflecting on what was going on in the group. The effects of fatigue and difficulties in holding on to concepts and memories also emerged.

I think the thing that happened to me is I reflect and suddenly I get tired and then I don't . . . The reflection is gone . . . and then I a little later can start again . . . but there's sort of something that stops, you know . . . in my mind.

Turid

We felt that it was a common experience in some groups for themes to disappear and then re-emerge much later on, perhaps with a different angle or perspective. However, with aphasia there is the difficulty in verbalizing what you are thinking when you want to, especially when those thoughts are abstract or new. Maintaining continuity of theme and content between sessions becomes doubly difficult.

Tom: *My assumption is that you need to be able to hold on to spoken information in order to be able to integrate it into memory, to be able to conjure it up again and re-think it, and reflect on it . . . what happens if that internal voice isn't there?*

Turid: *But I'm feeling often that the voice, internal voice, it is in your head but I can't tell you, and I think a lot of certain things that I can't tell you, but it is there . . . And certain things suddenly start and then goes . . . you know, I think aphasia is very bad for people in that way, because they can't talk straight away.*

We discussed the issue of collective responsibility in groups. Although the style and presence of a group facilitator does seem to have a demonstrable effect on group dynamics, we felt that each of us as group participants have a personal responsibility to contribute and support other group members. Negotiation, compromising and decision making as well as conflict resolution have as much to do with the participants as the facilitator. If a group doesn't go well, we all share in the responsibility.

The thinking comes from both of us . . . Both of us have to think.

Turid

Being a group facilitator

Our beliefs about how groups should be run differed initially and influenced the roles we adopted as group facilitators. The assumption in speech and language therapy training seemed to be that if you were competent at working with individuals, you could transfer those skills to groups, which implicitly were viewed as a collection of individuals. At the start of Tom's career, group work focused on individual communication skill-building within the group. This led to a focus on product and outcome, and a more didactic style of facilitation similar in many ways to one-to-one therapy. It also minimized intergroup interactions except those that fitted clearly with the transactional communication aims of 'getting the message across'. It fitted with an important underlying belief in the 'professional expertise' of the therapist as paramount.

I remember going to the group feeling uncomfortable, and maybe it was my anxiety . . . I then started to take on a persona of taking control . . . so I took over . . . And also, at least I perceived, there was an expectation from the group members that I would do that, that I would just run things . . . they let me do it, I did it!

Tom

From the outset, the psychotherapeutic approach seemed to be much more about creating the conditions for personal challenge and change in groups. This did not involve imposing an agenda or trying to solve problems, but rather listening carefully and reflecting back issues. For group facilitators this was underpinned by experiences in training of being a member of a psychotherapy group and of participating in individual psychotherapy.

The therapist is different from everybody else . . . but you're not the boss . . . it's still trying to get it even . . . The thing about me in the therapy is that I only say something if it is helpful but what I really want people is to think by themselves . . . I don't really like just . . . I was thinking when I saw you and you had that group, you sort of helped . . . we had agenda, but once you set it we could go on with it whatever we want to do really.

Turid

This style of being a group facilitator has implications for the type of support needed. For some therapists it can be stressful not to be able to set and control the agenda. Working in a group where the group participants have more say in the content and direction of the group can often be physically and mentally challenging. There is the potential for more conflict, as well as greater personal changes.

The nature and extent of clinical supervision in speech and language therapy and psychotherapy appear to be very different. Group psycho-therapists view themselves explicitly as a part of the group, not immune to the developing issues and relationships. Being aware of their integral involvement and having a place to reflect on their personal reactions is an important part of professional and personal development.

My style of facilitation changed if I felt anxious . . . I'm pretty sure that I became much more controlling . . . a way of dealing with my anxieties by shutting down the possibility of being challenged or the possibility of things not going to plan . . . so became much much less flexible.

Tom

I thought that [personal individual psychotherapy] was very helpful . . . not being so defended about everything, you know, and being a bit positive about my life and how I think other people.

Turid

The key issue of being a reflective practitioner started to dominate our discussions around what competencies a good group therapist needed. We agreed that having techniques up your sleeve to manage different group participants was useful, as were ways of planning groups, selecting group members and starting and ending groups, and so on. However, we seemed to have come to the same point in our thinking about group therapy over our years as group therapists, despite starting in very different places. Psychotherapy training and supervision foregrounded active self-reflection, and led on to skills development.

Whereas for me I think it was the other way round, so that I for lots of reasons wasn't particularly reflective and my training didn't encourage a lot of reflection . . . it felt to me like I was learning rules, but without really thinking about the why and how . . . I went on to question those rules and also started questioning myself . . . it's a different way round.

Tom

We felt that our attitudes about professional roles and practice as group facilitators stemmed from deeper underlying assumptions about who our group clients were, and consequently what they could and couldn't (or even shouldn't) do. If we felt that our clients were in some way incompetent, then we would want to shield them from taking on what we perceived to be difficult or dangerous roles. Therefore, if the facilitator felt that there was potential for unsafe choices to be made they would assume ultimate decision-making power rather than leave it to the clients. Equally, topics or situations in which strong emotions might be elicited would be avoided so as to protect vulnerable or labile clients. If, on the other hand, the facilitators viewed group members as competent adults, this would change the style of facilitation and communication radically.

Group therapy with people with aphasia: the road less travelled?

Origins

Group psychotherapy grew during World War Two as a result of a short-age of trained people to provide individual therapy. Over time therapists began to see that groups offered unique therapeutic possibilities. Inter-actions between group participants were seen as being instrumental in bringing about change. These interactions provided qualities not found in individual therapy, such as peer support, challenging, modelling and caring. Within a group people were able to test out new skills, gain new knowledge and perspectives, and begin to apply some of that new knowledge (Corey and Corey 1997).

Group therapy for people with aphasia evolved at roughly the same time, particularly in the United States. Again it was seen as a practical way of addressing the needs of a large number of armed service veterans with head injuries returning from World War Two (Kearns and Elman 2001). Since then there has developed a wide body of literature outlining different approaches to aphasia group therapy with a focus on psycho-social issues, family support, conversation and problem solving as well as communication and language (Elman 1999; Pound *et al.* 2000).

Complexity and challenge

In our experiences of being group participants and facilitators, the issues and goals arising in groups have been more complex and interrelated than some of the research might suggest. Aphasia impacts on communication, identity and lifestyle. Although different groups we have worked in have foregrounded each of these parameters differently at different times, they have all been present to a certain degree. Although flexibility is key in responding to a group's issues, it has also been helpful for us to be as clear as possible from the outset what the focus and format of a particular group might be.

The skill mix and resources necessary for exploiting the potential of groupwork may be beyond the scope of what some services want or are able to offer. Setting up a group that foregrounds identity issues while supporting communication could require skills in counselling and group facilitation, as well as knowledge of how to support individuals' com-munication. The group facilitator may also need supervision to deal with the range of emotional issues that can arise in such a group. Where a service is unable or unwilling to access these resources this should con-strain what is offered. Without careful consideration in advance of the skills necessary it is likely that a group facilitator will end up 'subverting' the focus of the group by redirecting it to fit their own skill base or comfort zone. However, an understanding of how groups work can have greater implications than therapeutic group work itself. This could legitimately be seen as part of wider continuing professional development in team and organizational management.

a degree of competence in the application of group principles can best be learnt through exposure to group psychotherapy and has importance within team-working and towards the understanding of organisational dynamics within institutions.

(Hull *et al.* 2000: 342)

Groups develop a dynamic that is more than the sum of the individual parts. Therefore, a firm grounding in group process is essential. This has implications for the wider training and support needs of therapists working in aphasia groups. Many therapists, however, have little additional training in group dynamics and process (see for example Kearns and Simmons 1985; Hamilton and Tracey 1996)

Yalom (1995) suggests that there should be four essential components in a training programme for group therapists:

1 observing experienced group therapists at work;
2 close supervision of their first groups;
3 personal group experience; and
4 personal psychotherapeutic work.

These latter two recommendations might be particularly challenging to the practice of most aphasia therapists but it is exactly those experiences that have brought about attitudinal and cultural shifts in our own practice as group therapists.

In working with groups, we would recommend careful thinking through of process issues. This might include:

* regular consideration of meeting place, time and duration;
* working to create a flexible, non-hierarchical and permissive environment where roles can be experimented with and skills developed;
* explicit thinking through of attitudes and assumptions about therapy and roles on the part of both group facilitators and participants;
* appreciating that whatever communication 'currency' participants use is relevant – not burdening people with verbals!

The mind is capable of restoring the brain, therefore exercising the mind in dialogue has a healing quality.

Turid

Aphasia therapists are increasingly recognizing the value of group therapy and of seeing the person with aphasia in a wider social and cultural context. Insights from psychotherapy can help us to see the value of thinking and reflecting, of process and context. The concept of a reflecting mind as distinct from the receiving brain is central to psychoanalysis and quite different in perspective to the predominantly medicalized language and thinking of many therapists working in rehabilitation. The cultivation of thinking and reflection with other minds is the primary objective of group psychotherapy. We believe that by combining this principle with the existing expertise of the aphasia therapist, groups can better promote authentic learning and change in everyday life. We are hoping that this can become a road more travelled.

References

Byng, S., Pound, C. and Parr, S. (2000) Living with aphasia: frameworks for therapy interventions, in I. Papathananasiou (ed.) *Acquired Neurological Communication Disorders: a Clinical Perspective.* London: Whurr Publishers.

Corey, M.S. and Corey, G. (1997) *Groups: Process and Practice* (5th edn). Pacific Grove, CA: Brooks/Cole Publishing Company.

Elman, R.J. (1999) Introduction to group treatment of neurogenic communication disorders, in R.J. Elman (ed.) *Group Treatment of Neurogenic Communication Disorders: The Expert Clinician's Approach.* Boston, MA: Butterworth-Heinemann.

Foulkes, S.H. and Anthony, E.J. (1957) *Group Psychotherapy: the Psychoanalytical Approach.* London: Penguin Books.

Hamilton, R.J. and Tracy, D. (1996) A survey of psychotherapy training among psychiatric trainees, *Psychiatric Bulletin*, 20: 536–7.

Hull, A., Haut, F., Rodriguez, C. and Cavanagh, P. (2000) Group psychotherapy: trainees' perspective, *Psychiatric Bulletin*, 24: 342–4.

Kearns, K.P. and Elman, R.J. (2001) Group therapy for aphasia: theoretical and practical considerations, in R. Chapey (ed.) *Language Intervention Strategies in Aphasia and Related Neurogenic Communication Disorders* (4th edn). Baltimore, MD: Lippincott Williams and Wilkins.

Kearns, K.P. and Simmons, N.N. (1985) Group therapy for aphasia: a survey of Veterans Administration Medical Centres, in R.H. Brookshire (ed.) *Clinical Aphasiology Conference Proceedings.* Minneapolis: BRK.

Pound, C., Parr, S., Lindsay, J. and Woolf, C. (2000) *Beyond Aphasia: Therapies for Living with Communication Disability.* Bicester: Speechmark.

Royal College of Psychiatrists (1993) Guidelines for psychotherapy training as part of general professional psychiatric training, *Psychiatric Bulletin*, 17: 695–8.

Swain, J., Finkelstein, V., French, S. and Oliver, M. (1993) *Disabling Barriers: Enabling Environments.* London: Sage.

Yalom, I.D. (1995) *The Theory and Practice of Group Psychotherapy (4th edn).* New York: Basic Books.

10

The Internet and aphasia: crossing the digital divide

Roberta J. Elman, Susie Parr and Becky Moss

Key points

- Many people with disabilities are not using the Internet much, particularly people with aphasia.
- Web design is often inaccessible and people with aphasia have trouble understanding the text on websites and finding their way around.
- This chapter talks about different ways to improve Internet access for people with aphasia. Many of the ideas come from a research group who looked at both web design and the way people tell their stories on Internet sites.
- This group were very sensitive to both the tone of a site and how easy it was to use.
- There are many ways to improve websites, for example, web designers could:
- make information more 'aphasia friendly';
  - provide communication support;
  - improve visual layouts; and
  - test visual icons beforehand to see if they are understandable.

The United States Department of Commerce reported that at the end of 1998 more than 40 per cent of Americans owned computers, with one quarter of those households connected to the Internet (US Department of Commerce 1999). The Department of Commerce also found that access to the Internet was associated with income, race, education and type of community. The profile of a household most likely to be connected to the

Internet was that of a white urban family having an annual income of at least $75,000. Those least likely to be connected were from young, poor, rural or minority households. The Department of Commerce report indicates that the 'digital divide' of the information rich and the information poor has actually widened compared to its survey in 1994.

Internet access for people with disabilities

People with disabilities are among the information poor. A white paper was commissioned by the National Science Foundation in the United States and presented at the Understanding the Digital Economy conference in May 1999, convened in response to a presidential directive (Waddell 1999). In this seminal paper, Waddell describes various laws and policies that affect those with disabilities being able to achieve adequate access to digital information. She states:

Unless the civil rights of America's 54 million people with disabilities are addressed during this period of rapid, technological development, the community will be locked out from participation on the basis of disability and the technological world will not be enriched by their diverse contributions.

(Waddell 1999)

Waddell's concept of 'participation' is consistent with that of the World Health Organization (WHO) in which participation is defined as 'involvement in a life situation'. WHO defines participation restriction as a problem that individuals experience in life situations when compared to individuals without disability who live in the same culture or society (WHO 2001). It is clear that many people with disabilities, especially those with aphasia, have participation restrictions with respect to the Internet and computer technology. Reducing such digital inequalities in the information age is a priority in UK health policy (Hughes *et al.* 2002).

Access to the Internet and other digital technology is critical. In the near future, people without Internet access will be extremely isolated and disadvantaged. It is expected that the Internet and related emerging technologies will impact the following activities among others: how we communicate, how we access information, how we receive medical care, how we learn, how we conduct business, how we work, how we conduct research and how we manage our government (Waddell 1999). Being on the wrong side of the digital divide will actually prevent full participation in life. Existing barriers must be overcome so that those with aphasia can achieve full participation in the digital economy. As Waddell states, 'The more the marketplace is transformed into a digital economy, the more obvious it is to the community of people with disabilities that they cannot participate due to inaccessible web design.' Waddell also states, 'Unless functionality solutions for accessibility are addressed today, the state of the digital divide tomorrow may be impossible to overcome.'

In this chapter, we describe initiatives regarding the promotion of Internet accessibility for people with disabilities. We start by discussing the applicability of general design standards to people with aphasia, then outline some studies that have specifically explored issues of Internet access for this group. We will focus, in particular on a study that was undertaken in London. Our emphasis will be on detailing the many barriers to Internet access that are faced by people with aphasia and on describing some solutions that currently are being considered.

Universal design standards

The Internet and information technology are transforming societies and markets at a rapid rate (Stewart 1999). However, inaccessible web designs are a significant barrier to those with disabilities. For people with visual impairments, graphical web pages may be inaccessible if screen or text readers cannot decipher images. For people with hearing impairments, web pages that contain sound clips or other auditory content are inaccessible without text captioning. Given these and other concerns, universal design standards for website accessibility have been discussed and published (Waddell 1998; Paciello 2000). There is a growing movement for website developers to use these standards in order to make all websites accessible to people with disabilities. Tim Berners-Lee, credited with being the inventor of the World Wide Web, states: 'The power of the Web is in its universality. Access by everyone regardless of disability is an essential aspect' (Brewer and Dardaller 1999).

Unfortunately, accessibility of existing websites for individuals with aphasia has not been specifically addressed as part of the universal design standards that are currently available. Two reasons may be that disability rights advocates are not aware of aphasia and those who are aware may not appreciate the disorder's full impact (Elman *et al.* 2000). In addition, those of us with knowledge about aphasia have not been present when such issues have been discussed with disability rights leaders and policy makers.

The issue of Internet accessibility could afford those affected by aphasia with a highly topical as well as visible venue from which to assert their civil rights while also increasing public and policy makers' awareness of aphasia (Elman *et al.* 2000). Disability rights rulings have determined that access to information and communication is a civil right for people with disabilities (Waddell 1999), an issue that is also reflected in the Disability Discrimination Act (1995) in the UK. Federal laws in the United States which include the Rehabilitation Act of 1973 (amended in 1986,

1992 and 1998), the Americans with Disabilities Act of 1990 (ADA), the Telecommunications Act of 1996 and the Assistive Technology Act of 1998, protect people with disabilities from discrimination in access to employment, commerce or information (Cook and Hussey 1995; Alliance for Technology Access 2000; Paciello 2000). People with disabilities, particularly those with visual impairments, have successfully used these laws to ensure their rights to information presented on the Internet (Waddell 1999; Paciello 2000). Lasater and DeRuyter (1999) point out that people with disabilities stand to reap the benefits of this new digital technology. However, it is obvious that unless this technology is made accessible, any potential benefits will go unrealized and will ultimately disenfranchise those who are unable to gain access.

Assistive technologies

There is a rich literature on assistive technologies for people with disabilities. Assistive technologies (AT) are defined as the 'broad range of devices, services, strategies, and practices that are conceived and applied to ameliorate the problems faced by individuals who have disabilities' (Cook and Hussey 1995: 5). Through AT, individuals with disabilities can be provided with increased access and function for life activities. Several technologies that might facilitate Internet access for individuals with aphasia are discussed below. The reader is directed to the AT literature for a more thorough discussion of philosophical issues as well as other products that assist people with disabilities in many aspects of living (Cook and Hussey 1995).

Barriers to access and aphasia

It is difficult to determine what the scope of the Internet access problem is for individuals with aphasia. Published research is not yet available. However, in an informal review of current websites, it is apparent that individuals with moderate or severe aphasia would have great difficulty in either comprehending page text or in placing orders for products. What does an accessible website look like for someone who has a moderate or severe aphasia?

Singh (2000) has addressed some of the linguistic, navigational and visual aspects that must be considered when developing a computer interface for those with memory or language limitations. He proposes development of an 'intelligent interface' to simplify computer use by addressing and modifying the following: query formulation, execution, and/or results; text manipulation, understanding and/or navigation; issues related to memory load; and analysis/classification of texts (Singh 2000).

Several recent research projects are investigating the ways we might make the Internet more accessible to people with aphasia. Sohlberg *et al.* (2002) received funding from the US Department of Education for a five-year project to create accessible electronic communication (email) for people with brain injuries. These researchers are adapting both hardware and software in order to allow people with cognitive impairments to use email. The project is also investigating how email can be used to re-establish social connections. Focus groups of individuals with brain injuries as well as their caregivers are providing feedback on various ways of adapting email for individuals with cognitive impairments. As part of the project, an on-line computer user profile and email client software are being created.

Pilot studies to date have revealed the following: the computer mouse needs to be modified or eliminated; limits need to be placed on computer keys to prevent excessive repetition; auditory and/or visual prompts are helpful for error detection; and interfaces need to be customized and individualized (Sohlberg and Ehlhardt 2001). The investigators are developing a 'think and link' user interface that allows the viewer to operate a simplified email system.

The MossRehab Email Project being organized by Linebarger is also addressing email accessibility issues for people with aphasia (Linebarger, personal communication March 2002). Linebarger and colleagues have developed a communication system in which each user records words and phrases in their own voice. By manipulating icons on a computer screen, the user can combine these recorded items to create longer utterances that they can then send as email attachments. These investigators are studying the use of this communication system with aphasia group members who receive weekly training in its implementation. Email messages are also being posted to a group website. Ultimately, the researchers are interested in investigating 'virtual' aphasia groups that could be hosted on the Internet.

Worrall *et al.* (2001) have also addressed Internet access for people with aphasia. Their AccessAbility grants project was funded by the Australian Department of Communications, Information Technology and the Arts. The investigators created student and instructor training manuals to increase Internet accessibility for people with aphasia. Twenty people with aphasia received accessible computers and local volunteers/tutors were recruited to assist them. Participants received approximately nine hours of training by the volunteers using the training manuals. Lessons covered such information as basic computer skills, screen and website navigation skills, search skills, locating and bookmarking website addresses and email skills. Pre- and post-test measures indicated that while some people with aphasia became independent Internet users, the majority of participants required continued support to access the computer and the

Internet. Worrall *et al.* have developed an 'aphasia-friendly' website to illustrate some design features for increasing Internet accessibility (http://www.shrs.uq.edu.au/cdaru/aphasiagroups/).

In addition, Worrall *et al.* have developed a set of guidelines for web development in collaboration with people with aphasia. It can be downloaded at http://www.shrs.uq.edu.au/cdaru/aphasiagroups/Download_Guidelines.html. The guidelines offer suggestions to website developers for improving access of web content, formatting and navigation elements.

Some detailed suggestions for improving website accessibility

Another project that is investigating website accessibility is currently taking place at Connect, the communication disability network, in London. The project, Inclusive Internet Technologies for People with Communication Impairment, is part of the Innovative Health Technologies Programme, and is funded by the Economic and Social Research Council and the Medical Research Council of Great Britain. The programme website is http://www.york.ac.uk/res/iht.

The project aims to address the issue of access to Internet technologies for people with aphasia. Every week for a year, a working group of 12 people with aphasia has met with researchers and engaged in a process of participative action research. One aim of the project was to develop a taxonomy of the barriers and facilitators that influence access to Internet-based technologies for people with aphasia. The group reviewed a range of websites, including those intended to be accessible to people with disabilities, those dispensing health related information and those explicitly concerned with aphasia. It also investigated chat-rooms, message boards and forums on various sites.

Detailed ethnographic notes formed the basis for building a prototype website (www.aphasiahelp.org) exemplifying accessible design, in close collaboration with the working group. The website was evaluated by other people with aphasia. The group has made preliminary comments about the purpose and audience of websites; language; supporting communication; information design, navigation and layout; images, graphics and text; and the purpose and audience of websites.

In the next part of this chapter, the barriers and facilitators identified by the UK group are discussed. This is work in progress and more detailed accounts of the findings will be produced in due course. However, in cataloguing the group's insights we hope to convey the diversity, complexity and subtlety of barriers to Internet access for people with aphasia and some of the ways in which these might be surmounted.

The purpose and audience of websites

- Some websites providing information about stroke and aphasia seem to be *about* people with aphasia rather than *for* them. The group is exquisitely aware of tone, style and language that excludes them, and has frequently commented on this: 'Obviously this other people you know not us but husband'; 'I don't think that's about us, the impression to me totally that is not about somebody like me. The second sentence, wow!' (The second sentence reads, 'Aphasia means an individual has difficulty retrieving words for speech and usually has some problems reading, writing and understanding spoken language.')
- The group has been demoralized by the inconsistency inherent in some websites which appear aphasia-friendly at the outset but contain links to academic papers, and fail to indicate the forthcoming change in style: 'It makes you feel even more foolish because you're trying to understand something and they're not letting you in on it. The rug is pulled from under your feet. You feel you're doing something for yourself by logging on, gaining control; this is almost like a big sign saying no, you can't come in here.'
- A particularly frustrating aspect of some websites has been the failure to provide a range of ways to contact them, other than the telephone: 'Why don't they have an email address as they're [communication disability charity] and they know the difficulties with speech and you can't – you don't have any access to telling them this?'
- The group has strong feelings about the need for websites to provide two versions of the same information. Group members like websites which provide short summaries of news stories, with the option to 'read more'. They feel this allows them to decide to pursue a story further or abandon it, a particularly useful feature when reading is difficult, 'What I think a good idea would be is people who've got limited reading just do a short passage for them, and then have a link of all the whole story, for people who can read a bit more.'
- The group feel that web designers could offer ways to convert information into an aphasia-friendly format, 'There ought to be two access points, one if you're someone with aphasia'; 'I would have thought maybe they could have the first page that comes up: would you prefer simplistic approach or can you tackle this, and if you click on "simplistic" it'd break it down into pages'; 'You can have this because some people read quickly you know? Press button then exactly same information different word.' With careful use this strategy could present information in a manageable style yet avoid editing out too much content.
- Group members become irked when the order of information on a website has clearly been arranged according to the priorities of the designer or the organization rather than those of the audience. One

group member, who was searching for a section on other people with aphasia, and was forced to scroll past a lot of irrelevant information first, said: 'I mean this – if you want – say if you want to go to centre to other people, not yet because board directors – no, mission statement – no, order t-shirt – no, so you have to . . . and then more. Like if you want to get in touch.'

Language

- Producing a precise URL can be problematic, and it is helpful when a web address contains relevant words. A member of the group wanted information about adopting a dolphin and found an appropriate website on her first attempt by typing www.adoptadolphin.com.
- Acronyms cause confusion; several members of the group have repeatedly failed to understand FAQ (frequently asked questions). Also problematic is word play which relies on being able to think about language in a certain way and understand double meaning. The group looked at a website with the URL '4dp' which stands for 'For Disabled People', one group member said, '4dp – why the devil should anybody look that up? That word that begins with a "d" [disabled] – at least that might mean something. Oh, I'd like to look at that, that would be much better.'
- Metaphor and abstract language were often interpreted literally by the members of the group. One website refers to 'dreams' when talking of hopes and ambitions, to which a group member responded, 'Why are they going to sleep?'
- On occasion suggestions have been misinterpreted as instructions because of use of the imperative voice, for example, 'Add this page to your favourites'. The group felt it would be useful for procedures which are optional to be clearly indicated as such, for example, 'Do you want to add this page to your favourites? If so, click here.' The phrasing of text within a link has also caused some problems of understanding what the link is for. For example, linking 'click here' to a long sentence of instructions is problematic.
- Jargon and complex vocabulary are best kept to a minimum. This is particularly important for websites where the content is about aphasia, and is aimed at people with aphasia. One group member found a website which used the word 'prevalent' in a quiz about aphasia, and remarked: 'What the hell is that?!'

Supporting communication

- Spelling accurately is often particularly challenging. While they still rely on a certain level of accuracy, search facilities which include a 'Do you mean?' query for misspelled words have received positive reactions. One group member typed 'anuarism' and the search was able to ask her: 'Do you mean "aneurysm"?' Predictive text could also reduce this difficulty and Singh (2000) suggests other assistive technologies for search facilities.

- Generating search terms proves to be difficult for some group members, both in terms of retrieving vocabulary initially, but also in narrowing the scope of a search. Semantic predictors may be useful for this task. Singh (2000) also suggests the negotiation of a search before the search is performed, for example, using icons to narrow the search at the beginning.
- Using message boards or site feedback forms the group members felt intimidated when invited to give comments with no supporting guidance or suggestions: 'I'm scared of this "comment". Because you have comment, but you can't express much. I can't, you know. I mean it's good, maybe help other people to do help through that. I know I have to say something but I can't.' They like to be provided with optional categories to complete if desired, 'because sometimes things just don't come out'. However, they feel it is excessive when numerous categories have to be completed before a form can be submitted: 'for [name of stroke charity] there's a lot of reading and writing, isn't there?!'; 'If I fill that thing on there it will take a long time for me to put together.' There is evidence of a tension between the desire to interact and fear that impairments will get in the way. This is compounded by a general lack of task support or examples on many web forms.
- The group has been particularly enthusiastic about websites with a colour selector, whereby users can change the font colour and background shade. Several group members feel this has a real impact on their reading ability, besides making the experience of a website more personal. These, however, also tend to be websites that have thought about accessible text and language. Such features provide opportunities for the user to control aspects of the site in a relatively straightforward way, which seems to lead to a greater level of engagement.

Information design, layout and navigation

- The visual separation of information that belongs together has caused problems. For example, spreading phrases or telephone numbers over two lines can be disruptive and confusing, especially when it occurs in menu panels where options are not delineated clearly through the use of borders or colour.
- Security or error messages in pop-up boxes often leave group members mystified: 'I get in a complete mess with these things. Work hard and hard and in the end you say yes, but is it yes or no?'; 'It's incredible. Several times I've gone to here and I press on one of those, and then I have to go back and back and forward again, so I can work out which one I have to press.'

- Likewise, help features of websites tend to be dense and incomprehensible. Both would benefit from less use of jargon and technical language, and simpler instructions. In addition, the help section requires users to read and remember step-by-step procedures; it would place fewer demands on users if help instructions remained on the screen throughout the help process, or if they were delivered in small sequential units as they are needed.
- A brief synopsis of what to expect from each menu category, triggered by placing the cursor over them in turn, has been found to reduce the need for aimless exploration of a website and thereby avoids the user getting lost.
- Blocks of text made up of short simple sentences with plenty of space between them are rewarding to read: 'Once you know it's in blocks they're nice just sort of short sentences, and you've got a space in between, so you think you've read rather more than you actually have.'
- Boxes which show all of the available options in a list are easier to use than drop-down lists. Finding 'United Kingdom' in an alphabetical 'select country site' list requires a lot of scrolling and some members of the group have found it extremely time consuming to read lengthy lists exhaustively. We have also witnessed people having problems manipulating the mouse to operate drop-downs effectively.
- Complex layout seems to have a negative effect. For example, multiple columns of text can be disorientating. Visual separation of different types of information (for example, navigation and content) helps, provided that each page on a site is laid out consistently. In addition, many people who have aphasia have had strokes that affect their right visual field. This means that information on the right hand side of the screen is often missed altogether.

Images, graphics and text

- Some font styles with narrow letters, such as Arial Narrow, are difficult to read because they look more cramped. Themed, florid fonts are also troublesome because letters are difficult to reconcile with their usual orthographic form; gratuitous use of capitals is problematic for the same reason. Large, broad, sans-serif fonts such as Verdana have produced the most positive reactions.
- Symbolic representations have been welcomed: 'I like that thing at the right, the drawing. I can understand what that is, it's about the brain problems and speaking problems'; 'It's effective, it makes sense immediately.' However, not all symbols and icons are clear and immediately understood, so such an endeavour should be approached with caution and with careful pre-testing.
- The group also liked pictures that directly support text: 'It's a break if you're reading, it sounds strange but to have something else.'

- Group members disliked moving graphics, however, particularly when there was no facility to disable the graphics: 'I'm not keen, it's distracting'; 'that receding heading is getting on my nerves'; 'I don't like this thing, constant moving picture, it's just annoying, like I can read that one [other text] but sometimes that gets in the way. I don't know why people do that. You can't stop it can you?'
- The group has been very sensitive to the images of disability presented by websites, and even fleeting, seemingly innocuous images have provoked strong reactions. They have criticized imagery that pathologizes disability: 'It's a horrible, like a hospital.' Overtly heroic images have also been criticized.

Moving in the right direction: some final suggestions and thoughts

There are no easy solutions for making websites accessible to those with moderate or severe aphasia. Given the varied expressive and receptive language limitations associated with aphasia, 'off the shelf' solutions are not currently available. However, numerous products have been developed to assist individuals with visual, hearing or mobility impairments, and to a much lesser extent those with cognitive impairments. Some of these commercially available products might be helpful in one or more ways with regards to Internet access for individuals with aphasia. The following examples are intended to be illustrative and do not comprise an exhaustive listing.

Enhancing Internet Access (EIA) was developed in Australia to assist individuals with cognitive or physical limitations. EIA includes a simplified web browser and a touchscreen with separate components for assessment and tutorials (Seiler *et al.* 1998). EIA appears to give users an introduction to the Internet via easier web browsing; however, it does not address the issue of page or text complexity once a desired website is located.

Another commercial product, Intellikeys®, is a touch-sensitive customizable keyboard that provides overlays (for example, pictorial representations or 'ABC' rather than 'QWERTY') to simplify text entry. It is possible that some individuals with a mild or moderate aphasia may be helped by changing keyboard configurations.

Finally, some individuals with superior auditory comprehension as compared to reading comprehension may be helped through use of screen readers. A screen reader converts text to synthesized voice output and is used primarily by individuals with visual impairments. The disadvantage for those with aphasia is that distortions in synthesized voice output may reduce auditory comprehension.

As previously stated, the complex issues related to barriers to the Internet for those with aphasia are unlikely to be solved solely through commercially available products. Instead, creative thinking must be used in order to develop both new products and new strategies to address the issues. One possible solution which could address the thorny issue of text complexity on the Internet would be for website creators to include photographs or highly iconic drawings whenever possible. Perhaps this idea should be discussed in context of the universal design standards that are currently available. Interested users would access a graphical interface by pressing a 'picture it' button on the website. Such graphical interfaces would also help others including those with reduced literacy skills or those speaking other languages. In fact a product that 'translates' text to graphical representations is now in the development stage (Paciello, personal communication January 2001).

A different type of model and potential solution is offered by the Speech to Speech relay service which has recently become available throughout the United States. This service, mandated by the Federal Communication Commission under the provision of Title IV (Telecommunications) of the ADA, enables people with speech impairments to place their calls through telephone operators. These operators have had special training in order to understand people with speech disorders or voice synthesizers. Operators relay the caller's message to the desired party by voicing it for them over the telephone. This service is funded through a nominal surcharge applied to all telephone users on their monthly telephone bills (Segalman, personal communication January 2001).

Through modification of a model such as Speech to Speech, one could envision training 'aphasia friendly' communicators who would 'interpret' website content for callers with aphasia. These trained communicators could access the same sites as the caller with aphasia through use of software products such as pcAnywhere® or WebEx® thereby allowing tandem on-line access for collaborative website browsing. The person with aphasia could then be assisted in navigating a website of their choosing with real time help from the trained communicator.

We must continue to work on the problem of how those affected by aphasia will be able to participate in our emerging digital technological world. Waddell envisions the following: 'Rather than creating a growing digital divide, emerging technology can enable full participation in the digital economy for everyone, regardless of age, disability or limitations of the technology available.' Campbell and Waddell (1997) suggest a need for 'electronic curbcuts'. We must partner with those affected by aphasia as well as those creating devices, standards and legislation in order to create digital curbcuts (or ramps) to ensure successful navigation through an increasingly digital world. Only then will those with aphasia be able to cross the digital divide.

References

Alliance for Technology Access (2000) *Computer and Web Resources for People with Disabilities*. Salt Lake City, UT: Publishers Press.

Brewer, J. and Dardaller, D. (1999) *The Web Accessibility Initiative*, World Wide Web Consortium, May (http://www.w3.org/WAI/#Guidelines).

Campbell, L. and Waddell, C. (1997) Electronic curbcuts: how to build an accessible website, *California Association on Postsecondary Education and Disability Communique*, Spring (http//www.prodworks.com/ilf/w5bcw.htm).

Cook, A. and Hussey, S. (1995) *Assistive Technologies: Principles and Practice*. St Louis, MO: Mosby.

Elman, R., Ogar, J. and Elman, S. (2000). Aphasia: awareness, advocacy, and activism, *Aphasiology*, 14(5/6): 455–9.

Hughes, K., Bellis, M. and Tocque, K. (2002) *Information and Communication Technologies in Public Health: Tackling Health and Digital Inequalities in the Information Age*. London: NHS Health Development Agency.

Lasater, J. and DeRuyter, R. (1999) The World Wide Web as a tool for practitioners and patients: a brief history and a road map for the future, *Topics in Stroke Rehabilitation*, 6(2): 66–72.

Paciello, M. (2000) *Web Accessibility for People with Disabilities*. Lawrence, KS: CMP Books.

Seiler, R., Seiler, A. and Ireland, J. (1998) Enhancing Internet access for people with disabilities, *Proceedings from Expanding Horizons, Speech Pathology Australia National Conference*, 49–55.

Singh, S. (2000) Designing intelligent interfaces for users with memory and language limitations, *Aphasiology*, 14(2): 157–77.

Sohlberg, M. and Ehlhardt, L. (2001) Email as a therapeutic modality. Paper presented to the American Speech–Language–Hearing Convention, New Orleans, LA, November.

Sohlbert, M., Fickas, S. and Todis, B. (2002) *Think & Link: Email for Individuals with Cognitive Disabilities* (http://www.think-and-link.org (accessed 17 June 2002)).

Stewart, T.A. (1999) The leading edge; A nation of net have-nots? *Fortune*, 140(1): 184–8.

US Department of Commerce (1999) *Falling though the Net: Defining the Digital Divide* (http://www.ntia.doc.gov/ntiahome/fttn99/contents.htm).

Waddell, C.D. (1998) *Applying the ADA to the Internet: A Web Accessibility Standard*, 17 June (http://www.irt.edu/~easi/law/weblas1.htm).

Waddell, C.D. (1999) *The Growing Digital Divide in Access for People with Disabilities: Overcoming Barriers to Participation*, Understanding the Digital Economy conference, 25–6 May (http://www.aasa.dshs.wa.gov/access/waddell.htm).

WHO (World Health Organization) (2001) *International Classification of Functioning, Disability and Health, ICF*. Geneva: WHO.

Worrall, L., Egan, J. and Schmidt, D. (2001) Barriers to learning the Internet for people with aphasia. Paper presented to the AccessAbility Workshop, May, Canberra, Australia (http://www.dcita.gov.au/commsconf/papers/linda.html).

Acknowledgements

Portions of this chapter were previously published as an article (Elman, R.J. (2001) The Internet and aphasia: crossing the digital divide, *Aphasiology*, 15 (10/11): 395–899. Reprinted by permission of Psychology Press, Hove, UK).

The Internet Project was funded by the Economic and Social Research Council and the Medical Research Council of Great Britain, as part of the Innovative Health Technologies Programme.

We would like to thank those who contributed to the Internet Project at Connect: Sally Byng, John Casburn, Margaret Chliatzos, Brett Garrett, Basia Grzybowska, Tony Moor, James Newbery, Leona Nicholl, Paul O'Donaghue, Tony O'Donnell, Tom Penman, Brian Petheram, Orah Schwartz, Becca Vinall, Jo Wauchope, John Wharton, Maggie Wilmot.

11

Directions without words

Monica Clarke with John Clarke

Key points

- This chapter illustrates how John and Monica communicate. It describes how they use gestures and drawings to talk with one another.
- John is very clear about what he wants to say and Monica is very good at guessing what John wants to say. But it isn't easy and it takes a lot of working through signs and clues and thoughts together.
- This story gives details about how John communicated to Monica that he wanted to take a trip to his old house in Slough.
- John and Monica have developed a picture system for supporting people to communicate. They include examples of the pictures and diagrams that helped them work out where John wanted to go.
- Monica says that people without communication problems have a duty to learn to communicate with people who have problems saying words.

It was a couple of days after that glorious Sunday at Camden Lock, and I was lying in bed giggling, thinking about Moses, when John pointed to the window. Then he pointed to me, then to himself. That meant he and I, outside something. But I was sleepy. And when I'm sleepy I reckon I have the right to sign off, to stop being forever the interpreter. I ignored John, closed my eyes, pretended to go back to sleep, and thought of Moses, about how OK he had left me feeling about this stroke and aphasia business.

I'd called him Moses because of his Jesus-sandals and ankle-length red gown. 'What a lovely life', he was saying, which had made me turn to look at him. He was bending down, level with John's wheelchair, back to me, long stringy blond hair hanging down between their faces. He swept his arms up and out, embracing the whole of Camden Lock with new age well-being and dangling copper bangles.

John agreed. Or rather, I think he did, for he was smiling happily, although he was shaking his head at the same time. The heady happiness of the housebound let out for a few hours had gripped him. A torrent of love gushed through Moses' long ginger beard as he bent down over my man's wheelchair, breathing past a silver nose ring into John's upturned face the stale Sunday morning smell of the Big Spirit. John opened his mouth. No sound. The words could no longer come. But the confusion of damaged brain and paralysed throat muscles went unnoticed by Moses, who put his head back and laughed, as if John had cracked the funniest of jokes.

Concerned, I started forward, as ever the careful carer, especially when other folk are around – hundreds of black-clad other folk at Camden Lock that Sunday morning. I went to stand by John's side. Protectively.

'Do you agree with me?' Moses was asking John, as his eyes swept up to mine, in an offer of friendship.

I remembered to find a smile. 'He can't speak, it's called aphasia', I was about to say, 'He's had a stroke, he . . .' I opened my mouth. I was desperate to explain, 'John can understand everything you say, but . . .' But Moses did not give me a chance.

'Foreigners!' he laughed, rolling his eyes to the rest of the universe as he came upright. Swinging his ponytail he hopped away, chuckling. John caught my eye. We laughed. He held out his good hand and grabbed mine. Does it matter if I can't speak, his grip said.

My step was light as I pushed his wheelchair back home. We giggled all the way. Suddenly John's inability to speak, read, write, walk, look after himself – suddenly his whole disability – seemed no longer so heavy.

We were just two people being different, as every other body at Camden Lock that Sunday morning had been different and that felt OK! I laughed out loud. The pleasure hung in front of my eyes as I watched John struggling to sit up in his bed, not able to reach the bedside trolley, which seems to have a direction of its own. I had to get up then, to move his urinals closer to him.

Again John gestured to the window, to me, to him. He was not going to let me get away with it this time. My heart sank. I knew what he meant. He wanted to go out somewhere. I had a meeting that afternoon. I had to prepare for it and I'd meant to stay at home to do this.

John looked at me intently. 'You wanna go out?' I asked the obvious. Yeah, he nodded.

'Somewhere in London?' A shake of the head. No. This meant travelling. 'Today?' A yes nod. My hesitant but not impatient frown was answered with a laugh.

'Can it wait?' He gave a half-hearted shrug. OK, so it is sort of important, I gathered. Anyway, by then the idea of driving out of London on a Tuesday morning did not sound like too bad an idea. It was early August (the week before the eclipse, I remember) and the weather was great that morning.

But where to? 'Where to, John?' Of course he couldn't answer this. 'Can you write it down?' I waited while he thought. After a few seconds he shook his head.

'To see Brian?' (his friend in Harlow). Shake of head. 'Your sister in Farnham?' Shake of head.

Luckily there are not too many people outside of London whom we visit, or places we regularly go to. It might be a park or something, I thought, maybe to Kew Gardens. 'To visit someone?' Shake of head. This was getting difficult. 'Is it far from London?' A pause while he thought. No. 'How many hours to drive there by car?' No reply, just a puzzled look. Silly girl, Monica should by then, after five years, know that he cannot not bring out a word in answer to a question.

'One hour's drive?' holding up one finger. Shake of head. Two hours, holding up two fingers? *Comme ci, comme ça* his open hand, palm down movement said. So-so. About two hours drive outside London, I murmured, mind searching north, south, east, west. I could not think of any place.

Meanwhile John was pointing to his wheelchair, that he wanted to get out of bed. As soon as I'd transferred him, he wheeled himself to his desk in the corner of the room. He hunted around in the drawer for a few minutes. Then he turned around, a photograph in his hand. His mother (dead long ago). 'Oh, to your brother's in Maidstone?' That was where his mum had lived when she died. No, John shook his head, still holding out the photograph.

'Could you show me on the map, John?' Yes. This time his nod was eager. He did not wait for me, but went straight for the map in the cupboard. I left him to it. It took him a few minutes to find the right page. I waited, watching him paging slowly through the big map book of Britain, thinking, they say then that you can't read, what are they talking about when I can see you seeing and understanding? But then I also know he can't read a line of text, we've tried this so many times and failed. How does this ruddy aphasia then work, I wondered, watching John, loving him, sharing his hard concentration with him. He was determined and I knew he would find what he was looking for. And he did. He pointed with his finger on the page and looked up at me.

'Slough!' I said. Yeah! he responded, this time with his voice, which comes out at exactly the right time sometimes, at the precise pitch, even though the sound was just a grunt, not a word. His eyes lit up happily. Slough is where he had spent his early years, before he was evacuated during the war. But that's a long time ago. Before my time.

Then his dream of the night before made sense. Very early that morning, when the sun was just brightening up the room, he had closed his eyes, while I was talking about something. Closed his eyes, a mystical smile on his lips. He had moved his head from side to side, while at the same time making circular movements with his hand, palm open in front of his face.

'You had a dream.' I'd been accurate for a change. He opened his eyes with a yeah look. Then he held his hand above his head. His sign for an adult person. Another of his *art words* as I call them. John has a self-created drawing-, gesture-vocabulary of about 20 or more art words, which he has taught us: family, friends, care workers, all of us. They have helped us to understand him so much better, because we have learned to use back to him his own gestures and drawings, mirroring them, repeating them, which has made understanding between us so much easier. We use his art words also when we speak to one another when John is listening, then he is included in more general conversation when we use his combination of drawing, writing, gesturing in John's way, the way he has taught us to do.

So his dream had been about an adult person, a shapely female figure, I could make out as he signed. (Thank God for the years of training he'd had in the pub with his mates, and their insulting descriptions of women.) Then his hand had gone down low, below his wheelchair. A tiny person. 'When you were a young boy?' A yes nod, followed by an arm movement. This, too, I understood, after a few wrong guesses. A swimming movement. It turned out that in his dream he had gone swimming with his friends, and his mum had been there with them, watching them.

'A happy dream?' Yes, his nod had said.

Now his dream made sense, the map still open in front of him. He was following a road with his finger around outer Slough, stopping at Stoke Poges. I noticed but did not really take notice. I was too busy thinking, *'oh, he says he knows where to go, huh.'* I was to regret this later.

But who did he want to go and see? Where exactly were we to go? I asked him and he grabbed a pen. He drew a building. 'A house?' Yes, with a nod. Number 13, he wrote (see Figure 11.1).

I had to trust this was the right number, for the very few things written down are not always accurate.

We arrived in Slough at half past twelve that afternoon. By half past two we were still driving around, with John almost remembering lots of times,

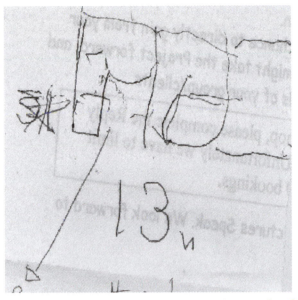

Figure 11.1   John drew this. They lived in house number 13 when he was young

then not, while I turned at one traffic light after another, right, then left, then around, checking each house number thirteen. We were becoming despondent. Afterwards I was to realize that when he had pointed left when we'd initially come off the M4 onto the A4 towards the town, and had changed his mind, neither of us trusting his instincts, that that was exactly where we were supposed to have turned off. That was the Stoke Poges road, where he had pointed to on the map that morning. Afterwards I wanted to kick myself for not believing that he knew what he was doing when he'd held his hand up above his head in the car and I thought he meant a big building and I asked 'a tower?' that I should have believed him when he nodded yes. Instead of which I stopped a man in the street and asked whether there was a tower in Slough and he said 'No, love, are you not talking about Windsor Castle?'

Afterwards it all fell into place. But during those two hours of driving around Slough it was all very confusing and so, so very insecure.

'We have to leave by three, John, I'm sorry', I said eventually when we pulled up outside yet another house number 13, disappointed, tired, disheartened. This time his shrug was one of defeat. Right then, though, we had to get back to London, back along the A4, past the university. Suddenly John gestured excitedly, saying with his hand go right, over the bridge. When we came over the bridge he made a sound and pointed left. About five hundred metres beyond the university, clearly rising above from behind houses and other buildings, during all those 50 intervening years, in red-bricked silence, stood the silo.

Wow! John had drawn it on another picture (see Figure 11.2) that morning. I had seen it, but at the time the silo had looked like a trumpet and I'd ignored that part of his picture, thinking that his mind was wandering. I had not asked what it was.

Go by car...

Over a bridge...

Past a silo!

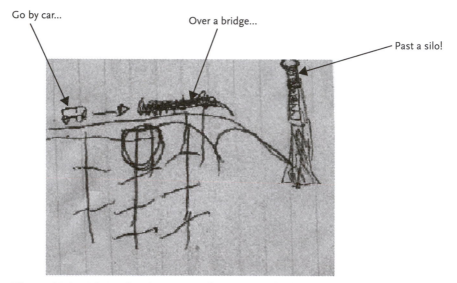

Figure 11.2 John's drawing giving directions to his house

We went there, past dilapidated, deserted factories. We were at last in the right area. When we passed the Horlicks factory the excitement in the car was so electric, it rippled up and down my arms.

'Did you walk over the bridge from your home to the factory?' (where he had worked when he was 16) – a can't remember shrug – 'or were you living on the other side of the bridge, John?' He could not remember. We were right there, I knew, but so far away. Then he made another swimming movement. The swimming pool in his dream again. I stopped and asked a lady in the street, 'Is there a swimming pool near here, please?' No, she said, looking at me funny-like. What John and I did not see was that we were in Pool Street then. I only noticed this later!

It was John who reached for the notebook in his bag, not me. It was he who took the pen and wrote LEE – then ended the word with a P. 'Leep Street?' I asked. No, he shook his head, now really confused. Then he put an S in front of the L. 'Sleep Street?' No. He took the pen and scratched the S out. That left us with Leep Street (see Figure 11.3).

'Tell you what I'll do,' I said. I was about to make my first intelligent suggestion for the day. 'I'll go and get an A–Z [map] of the area. Then we

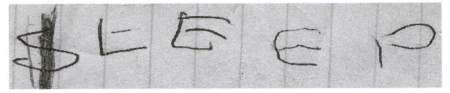

Figure 11.3   John wrote this

can look for Lee-something Street.' As I was paying for the map I had the sense to ask the lady whether there was a Lee-something Street in the area?

'Leeds Road,' she said immediately. 'Second street on the left,' she said and my heart sang. 'Just past the small roundabout', she said.

The house was exactly where John had drawn it that morning, the third one in the street. Number 13. What joy! He'd found it. And it sat smack bang between Pool and Stoke Poges Lane as well. We sat outside in the car under an all-knowing sun for a long while, staring at the freshly painted house with newly double-glazed windows and fresh net curtains. To stop John from pointing as his unspoken memories flooded out in excited gestures, I promised that we would return there soon, for we really had to get back to London.

We were on such a high as we came back, it seemed as if the car's wheels were gliding over the M4 without making contact. The motorway cleared itself so we could move by unhindered, as friends do for each other when they share a happiness. And then what did John do when we got home? For a long time he sat studying the map of the area which we had bought in Slough. The map, which includes the areas of Slough, Maidenhead, Windsor and Eton, is huge. I did not know what he was doing, what he could recognize, what he could or could not read. Yet when I saw the map later, there from among hundreds of streets, I saw that he had located and put a circle around Leeds Road (Figure 11.4). I should not have been amazed to see a swimming pool a finger-length away.

What an amazing day. John's sister phoned later that week. I'm so glad I had not asked her the address of their family home before we had set out. I told her John had taken me to Slough to their old house.

'Oh, number 13 Leeds Road,' she said, quite matter of factly.

John has died since I wrote the little story above. Before he died, John and I started a project called Pictures Speak, teaching others how to support communication if their work involves people with communication difficulties. We noticed that people in wheelchairs are given wheelchair ramps to use. But we also noticed that hardly ever is someone with a communication difficulty given a communication ramp. This is unfair and unequal, we reckoned.

So we started to teach people how to build communication ramps. We

Swimming pool

Leeds Road

Pool Lane

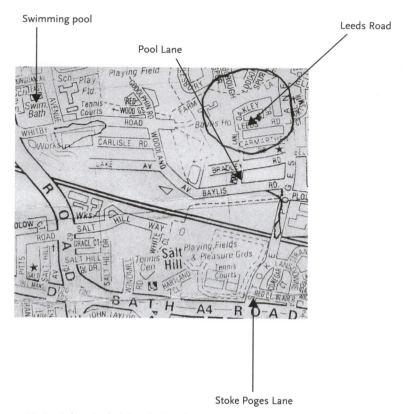

Stoke Poges Lane

Figure 11.4 John circled Leeds Road

felt that as John had the communication difficulty, he was the best person to do the training and as I was living with him, I was the best person to help him. So we invited other people with aphasia and their carers to join us.

We train health and social care workers how to support communication. We work with communication support trainers. We are supervised by local speech and language therapy services. We feel our abilities are utilized and recognized because instead of just being asked to 'tell our story' we are an important part of the team giving communication support. This is how Pictures Speak started.

John was still in the acute hospital after his stroke. I remember how worried he was, how worried both of us were, because it had dawned on us that not only had he lost his speech, but he could no longer read. Nor could he write. He was ill. I felt helpless. Every time I asked him how it was going, he would just shrug a 'what's the use' shrug. So one day I went out and bought a kiddy's paint set and drawing paper and left it by his bedside to give him something to do, because there was no television to watch in the ward either.

That started him painting. He'd been drawing and painting ever since then. Everyone, including the staff at hospital, saw and admired his work.

When he was discharged from rehab I packed his paintings and drawings into a big plastic bag and took them home. And forgot about them. Four years later I opened the bag.

'Hey, this looks good', I said about the drawing of two figures (Figure 11.5). 'What does this mean?' I asked. 'You drew it long ago, in 1995.'

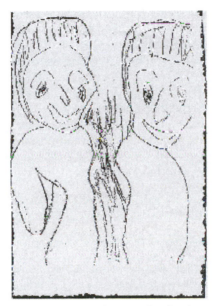

Figure 11.5   Two figures. Drawn by John shortly after his stroke

John smiled. He pointed to himself and then to me. Him and me. Then he frowned and took the picture from me. Putting it on his lap he pointed to the dark bit in the middle, between the two figures. Shaking his head, he looked up at me from his wheelchair. A real sad look.

'Does this mean you were sad about something when you drew it?' I asked. Yeah, he nodded, moving his finger up and down over the dark bit between the two figures, frowning deeply. Then he made a swinging movement with his good arm, from small to large. A widening gap.

'Ah!' It dawned on me. 'You were worried about us – that we would split up?' Yes, he nodded. 'Are you still worried about that?' Another nod. 'But why, when we're still together?' John pointed to his genitals and to mine. And at the picture, the bottom bit. The figures in the drawing have no bottoms.

'By golly, John. You mean you've been worried all this time that you and I were going to split up because we're not having sex?' Now the nod was very slow, his lips pursed in anger. 'And you were telling us about it in the picture, but nobody was listening!'

I felt like kicking myself. I still do. Neither I, nor any of the speech and language, occupational or physiotherapists (and there had been many) had spoken to John about his fears, which were plainly to be seen in his paintings and drawings strewn all over his bed and locker all those months. Not even the resident psychotherapist on the rehab ward (who at the time felt there was no need for her services as John had not 'asked' for counselling) had noticed. We had been too busy trying to get him to say words, to brush his teeth, to re-learn to make tea, to transfer, to walk. All important things. But no more important than his non-verbalized fears. Nobody had been listening. All of us were ignoring him when he was speaking through his pictures – trying to start conversations through his drawings.

So, John and I started Pictures Speak, to make sure that those involved with people who have communication difficulties – in hospital, in the community, at home – would realize how important it is that those of us without communication difficulties have a DUTY to learn to communicate effectively with those who have difficulty using words. Since John died I have carried on with this work.[1]

Note

1 If you would like to know more about the training programme for health and care workers, please contact Monica at monicaclarke@freenet.co.uk

12

Time please! Temporal barriers in aphasia

Susie Parr, Kevin Paterson and Carole Pound

Key points

- Many disabled people find it difficult to get around: getting into buildings and using public transport.
- Narrow doorways, no lifts, no ramps: space can be a problem. How space is organized disables many people.
- But for some disabled people, especially people with communication disability, time, rather than space, is the problem.
- In this chapter the authors talk about how speed is important in our society and the ways people with aphasia find communication difficult especially when they are under pressure to be quick.
- Research and stories from everyday life show that taking longer to communicate can cut people off from work, social contact and humour.
- The authors talk about trying to find ways of reducing time pressures on communication.
- Sometimes this means changing the way people work, services are planned and organizations are run.
- The authors say disabled people have a right to get into places and use services in our society and they also have the right to do things at their own pace.

Time,
Time,
Time, see what's become of me
While I looked around for my possibilities.
                    (*A Hazy Shade Of Winter*, Simon and Garfunkel 1966)

Time plays a central role in our lives. In the developed world we are told that 'time is money' and 'time is of the essence'. We must save time, not waste it or fritter it away. Some of us are cash rich, but time poor. We are enticed by fast cars and food, and high speed Internet connections. We are under pressure to be efficient, to produce something or to perform a task in the shortest possible time. Tasks – or people – that take up too much time are associated with negatives like waste and delay (Adam 1995).

Although the time pressures at work in day-to-day life seem to be an unavoidable feature of Western post-industrialized culture, this taken for granted reckoning of temporality has many negative impacts, such as stress and burn-out. For people with communication impairments who struggle with time and timing in everyday interactions the impacts of temporal norms and expectations can be profoundly excluding, as we hope to show in this chapter.

Our ideas are theoretically grounded in the principles of the social model of disability (see Tregaskis 2002 for a current overview of the theory). The social model represents disability as being socially pro-duced rather than as an inevitable result of impairment (UPIAS 1976; Finkelstein 1980; Oliver 1983, 1990). This perspective challenges the individualized and medicalized model that frames disability largely in terms of cerebral and anatomical 'abnormalities'.

According to the social model, individuals are not disabled because they have an impaired body or mind. Rather, they are disabled because the contemporary organization and norms of society neglect their needs and rights, thereby placing barriers in their way. Thus, from the social model perspective, disability is a human rights issue rather than a medical and therapeutic problem: disabled people face a particular form of oppression and institutional discrimination (Barnes 1994).

The key tenet of the social model is that disability is a social restriction imposed on people with impairments. To illustrate, a wheelchair user is denied access to spaces and places not because they cannot walk, but because of a failure to recognize the mobility needs of people other than those who are ambulant. The cause of the problem is located outside the individual and squarely within the spatial environment. Likewise, a person with a visual impairment is disabled by the lack of audio alerts, tactile surfaces, good lighting and colour contrasting. A person with a hearing impairment is disabled because induction loops, minicoms and trained signers are not available. A person labelled as having a 'learning disability' is disabled by restrictive definitions of competence and responsibility. A person with communication impairment is not disabled because they cannot keep pace with conversation, but because the framework for social interactions fails to accommodate their temporal style of communicating.

In this chapter we reflect on the hidden ways that time pushes and pulls on everyday life and explore how it impacts on the experience of people with communication impairment, in particular those with aphasia. We consider how temporal rules and norms concerning communication contribute to the social exclusion of people with aphasia. We will examine this process of exclusion from the world of work and social interaction and service delivery.

Our reflections are informed by our perspectives as a theorist (KP), therapist (CP) and researcher (SP) living with and/or working in the field of communication impairment. We draw on a number of sources including in-depth interviews exploring insider perspectives on aphasia (Parr *et al.* 1997) and an on-going ethnographic study of the experience of people who have severe aphasia (Parr 2003). In the latter project, people who struggle to communicate in any form agreed to be observed in a number of different situations and settings, including nursing homes, day centres, shops and hospitals, and to talk about their day-to-day lives. In addition, close family members and in some cases institutional carers talked about their experience of living with and assisting people with severe language impairment.

We also draw on experiences of everyday interactions between people with and without aphasia who come to Connect – the communication disability network centre in London. Insights from communication in social, work-orientated and therapeutic interactions illustrate how time is a key player in the social construction of disability.

Social model theory and time

Initially those promoting a social model focused mostly on inaccessible design and management of social, cultural and physical space as a source of social exclusion. Social model theory has highlighted and challenged the barriers and obstructions in public and domestic space that bring about disability (Zarb 1995; Imrie 1996; Freund 2001).

The growing strength and orthodoxy of the social model of disability has been helped in no small part by theorists and activists refining and extending their understanding of the disabling environment to include people with differing impairments. While the removal of spatial barriers is an important component in the emancipation of disabled people, other barriers such as temporal ones have been less emphasized. However, Sally French (1992) – referring to people with visual impairment, and Mairian Corker (1998) – referring to people with hearing impairment, have both highlighted the disabling nature of time, and the fact that the re-arrangement of social space is not always the answer to every problem faced by disabled people. In addition, others have argued that the social model's successful politicization of space should be accompanied by a critical politics of time (Paterson and Hughes 1999; Paterson 2001).

Aside from these contributions, time has been considered not in terms of disabling day-to-day dynamics, but in terms of the ways in which temporality is determined by social and economic changes between historical periods. The impact of these changes on the treatment of disabled people shows how time is a powerful excluding force. Mike Oliver (1990) and Vic Finkelstein (1980) have both raised the issue of time when arguing that disability is produced by historical changes in the social and economic conditions of society. They argue that the Industrial Revolution played a significant part in the exclusion of people with impairments by changing the pace of social and economic life (see also Gleeson 1999).

Prior to the growth of factory production, disabled people were not segregated from their community since the pace of peasant life was slower and work was less pressured. Time was not kept by clocks, but was understood in terms of natural rhythms such as the passage of the day and the growing of crops. Activities were tailored to a peasant's own capabilities and tasks lasted as long as the job required (Thompson 1974). People with impairments were able to work on the land and play an active role in the small cottage industries, at their own pace. However, the development of the mechanized production line established new ways of working. Time-keeping and standardized production rates stigmatized the speed of people with impairments in the workplace. As industrialization took hold, the rhythm of the mechanized factory floor dominated the rhythms of nature and personal working style. The pace was set.

These new working conditions made people with impairments appear slow, and they started to be classed as 'unfit', 'unable' and 'disabled'. As a result, disabled people were reconfigured, treated as a social problem and placed in institutions (Oliver 1990; Finkelstein 1980). The commodification of time and the established rule of clock time are now the taken for granted backdrop for our daily lives. As such, speed is worshipped, adored and venerated (Adam 1995).

Not just bricks and mortar: time and communication impairment

Speed, valued for its own sake, can impose different types of problems and limitations on people. If individuals cannot (or will not) keep up with the 'need for speed', then they are left by the wayside: they are excluded and discriminated against. As Adam (1995: 101) argues 'the link between speed, economics and clock time operates against the principle of equal opportunity, whether this be in relation to different sexes, occupational groups, cultures or categories of people'. Disabled people are clearly one such category of people disadvantaged by the time economy.

Let's consider how temporal norms can disadvantage people with communication impairment. This is most immediately apparent in personal interaction. Conversation can take a variety of forms (small talk, chat, discussion, gossip and so on). Each has a specific timescale for participation based on the communication style of non-disabled people (Paterson and Hughes 1999; Paterson 2001). There is what might be described as an etiquette of timing that structures everyday social encounters.

If one's speech or language is slow with respect to these temporal conventions then one is judged incompetent and what is said is devalued. For example, imagine an individual with language impairment, who requires that their communicative partner devote more time to listening to what they are saying. This person is at a disadvantage because there is no room for manoeuvre in the time margins when negotiating social encounters. One must keep in sync with the tempo and pace of conversation. Any interaction that flouts these conventions is viewed as an embarrassing failure. People with communication impairments are often excluded from conversation and chit chat because the etiquette of these situations does not allow them the time to express what they wish to say. As Wendell (1996) points out, the taken for granted nature of the rhythms and pace of everyday life help to bring about disability.

In the remainder of this chapter, we attend to problems that are constituted predominantly by the taken for granted tempo, pace and rhythm of everyday life and explore how these relate to the experience of people with aphasia. Reflecting on the social exclusion of people with aphasia, we describe some ways of dismantling temporal barriers.

Aphasia and time

I'm sorry my stroke and speaking slowly . . . um . . . talking slow.

Sharon

Please, I've had a stroke. I'm aphasic and have problems. Can you speak very very slow? And they end up me and them practically arguing on the phone to slow down and I go: 'I am aphasic' and that confuses them because they haven't got a clue what aphasic is. And then it always is: 'Oh yes, my aunt had a stroke' or 'My uncle had a stroke.' 'Oh isn't that a shame?' And I'm not even worried whether it's a shame and I go: 'Oh never mind, never mind, never mind.' And I come off the phone maybe three quarters of an hour after and I go: 'Well why do I have to worry about this? It's costing me money on the telephone.'

Alf

Well once I threatened to complain. I told them that if they . . . if they . . . I've forgotten what it was about now. I said I was . . . I was writing to the prime minister about this. Oh very blasé, blasé, and she said 'Oh are you?' I'd take all day about it and do it all . . . all in my . . . mmm, mm, and write it again and again until I . . .

Martha

Sharon, Alf and Martha are talking about experiences that are common-place for people who have aphasia and for people with other communi-cation impairments. Sharon apologetically explains to people she meets that her speech is slow, as she searches for the correct words to convey her meaning. Alf's aphasia means that it is hard for him to understand what people are saying. He can understand if they talk slowly, but this is difficult to explain and the time taken to make his point and clarify his situation ends up costing him money. A former doctor, Martha, also experiences difficulties talking and understanding but, like many people with aphasia, she also struggles to read and write, and knows that any such activity will cost her a lot of time and effort.

But the influence of temporal conventions is felt beyond personal interaction. Levels of participation in a fast paced social world frequently rest on the ability of services, structures and people to accommodate different temporal frameworks for communication. Sharon, Alf and Martha's experiences suggest this sort of temporal accommodation is a rare occurrence. Nowhere are time pressures felt more keenly than in the world of work, a world from which people with aphasia are commonly excluded.

Aphasia, time and work

Trawling the in-depth interview transcripts for mention of problems associated with time and timing, it is striking how many people linked this issue with their struggle to get back to work. Only one out of the 50 people interviewed (30 of whom had previously been in work) was able to return to employment full-time following the onset of aphasia. For Kiran, speedy reactions to what others said or did were essential in his work as a senior teacher. Although he has returned to the school environment he loves, it is in the capacity of part-time classroom assistant:

Obviously I cannot manage kids. I know that now. In that I tend to take slightly longer than most teachers and adults do in reacting to a given situation. By the time I react, the incident is over. In my present post, I can see teachers making sometimes the wrong decisions for the children, but as a classroom assistant I have to keep my mouth shut. I'm perfectly capable of making decisions, but I can't have too many ideas at once.

Similarly, Emma (who worked in a bank in Chicago prior to her stroke) reflects on the rapid pace of her communication in the workplace prior to aphasia. She cannot contemplate returning to the same kind of work now, partly because of her slower pace.

I'm not a fast-speaking person. Um . . . I've got a little bit of a problem, but, you know . . . well I was ever so fast in my job and speaking as well.

For Andrew, who used to work manufacturing surgical instruments, the experience of stroke and aphasia at the age of 49 was traumatic: 'like hitting somewhere at 100mph. Oh I was absolutely shattered.' Andrew could barely speak at all in the beginning and he struggled to follow what others said, as he explains when talking about the consultant who was looking after him in hospital:

I guess one day he did come round to some of the staff because . . . I don't remember the words. I couldn't speak you see. No way of communicating and er . . . er . . . he would start talking but he was talking to me . . . er . . . er . . . more quickly. I couldn't understand what he was . . . Um . . . slowly, slowly . . .

When he is talking about the social impact of the stroke, Andrew uses metaphors concerning speed and timing. This is particularly the case when he describes his male colleagues' reaction to his illness and his feeling of being unable to keep up with them. His comments underline the competitive aspects of contemporary working life: '*Male friends couldn't talk and the er . . . they were sympathetic. I was this. You're in a race and you fall over.*'

Interestingly some people with aphasia talk of the relief of leaving behind the stresses of full-time work and the pressures imposed by increased demands and shrinking resources: '*Having my stroke has made me realize what I can and cannot do . . . that's not an easy thing to realize when nothing like this has ever happened to you*' (Connect group member).

Like many disabled people, some people with aphasia do find opportunities to re-engage in work, largely by negotiating terms and conditions that accommodate changes in their levels of health, energy and speed. Often these negotiations concern temporal barriers. For example, additional time may be needed for travelling, particularly if the person has a motor impairment. Equally people with aphasia may have to negotiate extra time for work that is dependent on language, for example, administration, writing up notes, making a telephone call or engaging in discussion and decision making.

However, many people with aphasia fall at the first hurdle unless the employing organization makes accommodations to temporal differences from the start. For example, job applicants attending an interview are usually expected to demonstrate their potential for employment within a tightly imposed time frame. They are expected to read and process written information (which may be inaccessible for a person with aphasia without interpretation) and complete application forms (again a timely process where communication support may be needed to translate thoughts into written form). If potential employers cannot adapt their temporal expectations at the outset, there is little hope of people with aphasia ever reaching the starting point of negotiating terms and conditions (itself a language and time-based process).

Commitment to inclusion risks becoming tokenistic unless the organization can respond creatively and flexibly to the alternative time framework which communication impairment encourages us to construct. At Connect we have found that the interviews involving people with aphasia (both as job applicants and as members of interviewing panels) take approximately three times longer than routine interviews. Preparation and follow-up time for such interviews is a prerequisite. This allows accessible material to be developed from existing documentation (such as briefing notes and job descriptions). Criteria for decisions about the post and terms of employment need to be negotiated, clarified and revisited with people who have aphasia, both before and after the interview. Interviewers or applicants who do not have aphasia need to be trained and equipped to communicate effectively with interviewees or panel members who do. This is another time consuming process. However, such an investment of time enables participation of people with aphasia and brings with it multiple benefits along with challenges.

With reference to the day-to-day organization of work, Sally French (1992) raises the subject of time as an equal opportunity issue. Although discussing people with visual impairment, she makes pertinent points about disabled people as a whole. She argues that there is a damaging belief that disabled people can be given equality at work simply by supplying them with the appropriate technological support. Of course, this can help some enter the labour market but it is unlikely to counteract the disabling effects of our adoration of speed. The neglect of this time factor means that disabled people are forced to sideline their own temporal needs and buy into the notion that the reorganization of the spatial environment will be the primary domain within which they are allowed to negotiate equal participation.

French asserts that people with visual impairment have to continually battle against the view that they are 'less able' than sighted people in their workplace since the tempo and pace of most jobs are designed to meet the needs of those with vision. Moreover, promotion is often based on the willingness to work above and beyond the requirements and hours of one's position. This means that many disabled people compete on an unequal basis because temporal conventions discriminate against them. They have to surrender a greater chunk of their personal time in order to appear as 'capable' as their non-disabled work colleagues (French 1992). We are arguing that these insights of French are pertinent to the experience of people with aphasia who are re-entering the workplace.

Aphasia, time and the social world

Andrew describes how his social relationships with work colleagues were affected by his difficulty in keeping up with the pace of work. Others confirm that the timing and pace of communication can profoundly affect their personal identity and can undermine even the most robust friendships. Betty, who was a writer before she had a stroke, describes how she finds it impossible to contribute to a local writers' group she attends. She often wants to add to the discussion but by the time she has the floor, she finds the thought she wanted to convey has gone: 'the moment has passed'. This experience (commonly described by many people with aphasia) makes her lose confidence and she has become increasingly reluctant to go out.

For Christopher, being visited by a friend has become a painful rather than a pleasurable experience. Christopher, who speaks very slowly and takes a long time to formulate his thoughts, finds that his friend is unwilling to wait for him to contribute to the conversation. The whole dynamic of their interaction has changed. Christopher finds their time together uncomfortable:

And he's kept coming along and I must admit I've been thankful to see him. But lots and lots of occasions . . . uh . . . I know that I can't. I know the fact that he tries. I think he's impatient. I presume because I'm not quick enough . . . because um because um . . . because he's got to have a reaction. Cos I want him to have the reaction which I used to be able to have. Before I was ill I used to have a constant repartee with him.

Like Christopher, others with aphasia are often exquisitely sensitive to the reactions of others and to their patience or lack of it: *'I feel that people are left thinking oh God I wish she'd hurry up.'*

People with communication impairments often place a greater value on the time of others than on their own time needs. Few see a communication breakdown as the failure of others to adjust to new time rules. The subtle shifts in timing required within this new communication dynamic are not easily acquired. Different temporal conventions in communication demand a lot of those who have aphasia and of those who do not. Not least the demands include a commitment to personal change and development and a willingness to handle uncertainty and failure.

Aphasia, time and humour

Language is the currency of friendship. We use language to chat, gossip, share secrets, express affection and concern and tell jokes. Language is a medium of humour, with timing a critical component in successful story and joke telling. Kiran became painfully aware of the impact of aphasia on the cut and thrust of humour with his friends. Before his stroke, humour was a critical part of his identity and also a means of expressing his friendship. Now his humour is inaccessible:

Oh God, my humour was really important. I used to talk it very fast. I have the humour still but I cannot talk it fast enough. I have to take it in. It goes all the way back into my files and by the time it comes out, it's too late. The conversation has changed. And that is the most . . . the hardest thing to accept. I get really really frustrated when two people are talking and I want to lighten it up with humour. And I cannot do so.

People with aphasia at Connect also comment frequently on loss of humour as an unhappy feature of their post-stroke identity. However, as time passes a new and different ability to engage in humour is often revealed. Many Connect clients develop techniques and draw on facial expressions, gesture, and physical props (people, objects, drawings and so on) in order to express humour. In addition, the timing of jokes is often stretched, allowing them to be developed and shared more gradually. Here, as in other social communication, the reallocation of time contributes to a process of engagement, revealing the potential for shared enjoyment and expression of identity.

Time together

Spending time with others who have aphasia or other impairments enables access to a world where different rules of time and timing are thankfully shared. Clients at Connect (where much group work takes place) value a context in which diverse styles of interaction are temporally accommodated. For many, developing and sharing new temporal conventions with others affords a welcome sense of familiarity, community, power and personal well-being.

However, managing the different communication and temporal styles of a group of people with diverse forms of language impairment is no easy matter. People (with and without aphasia) who work as communication facilitators within conversation groups have commented on the challenges of orchestrating enjoyable, inclusive conversation in the context of different and highly individual, communication styles.

Uncontrolled pace, silence and other communication 'trouble spots' in group conversation, if unmediated, can have a significantly negative impact. When there is a lengthy period of uncertainty (for example, if the group are trying to work out what one member is expressing) there is a risk that the thread of conversation will be lost. More and more people may lose the plot, and confusion ensues. The opportunity to focus on a conversational topic and explore it in some depth is easily lost:

When that happens . . . I can't do that, the summary thing . . . my head can't hold it and say it again.

(Connect group member)

Similar problems arise when one group member dominates the air-time. People, with or without aphasia, who communicate fluently may gain the upper hand in conversation. Faster, more fluent access to language affords power while hesitancy and pauses to frame ideas and translate them into words can result in opinions and voices being silenced.

When any communication constitutes a major struggle, those living with people who have severe aphasia find the rhythms and routines of their lives are changed. Negotiations and decisions are no longer easily conducted and sometimes become a protracted process of probing, checking out and trying to guess what is meant. Such episodes occurred many times during the observational sessions with 20 people who have severe aphasia. Sometimes it could take up to 15 minutes to establish the point that the person with severe aphasia was trying to make, and often the struggle would be abandoned and the point lost because it was taking up so much time. Any such process demands considerable ingenuity and stamina on the part of a conversation partner, and may be helped by in-depth knowledge of the person concerned, as this excerpt, describing a conversation between Mr Fell and his wife, demonstrates:

Musical? Light opera? Gilbert and Sullivan?' she queries. 'No, no.' 'Write it down for me. I'm not sure what you're trying to say.' 'Um, um, um.' He looks up and waves his pen around. 'Carry on writing down.' He has a pen and pad on the bed-table in front of him. The pad seems quite high up and quite far away from him. It looks awkward because he has to sit forward to write. She stands to one side (his right) and looks down at what he is writing. 'To do with the band?' 'No.' 'To do with yourself?' 'No.' 'To do with singing?' 'No.' 'Conducting?' 'NO' (very loud). She continues, 'Alright, try and tell me.' He indicates his right side, says: 'Um um,' and stares around. He holds the pen in his left hand. 'To do with yourself?' He points to his left. Then suddenly makes a curving movement: clearly holding and turning a steering wheel. 'Driving?' 'Ahhh, mmm!' He nods and smiles, looks relieved. 'Home Care . . . you used to drive for Home Care?' 'Mmm.'

Although there are ways in which conversation with people who have severe aphasia can be supported (for example, using drawing or writing, checking back that you have understood the person's meaning correctly), this process in itself takes time and can disrupt the natural flow of interaction. Supporting someone's conversation while walking along is particularly difficult because useful props are not to hand. Supported conversation needs dedicated time, a table, pens, pencils and paper and sometimes resources such as maps and pictures all of which take time to organize. Physical and social environments which provide such conversation ramps (Kagan 1998) are rare in health and home settings. The person with aphasia and their communication partner may need to take responsibility for negotiating the extra time and energy required to support communication.

The husbands, wives and partners of people with severe aphasia describe the time dedicated to communication, trying to understand what their partner is expressing. And it's not just the difficulties of immediate communication, but trying to piece together evidence and information, for example, when the person is ill. Gathering clues, checking out, thinking back on the sequence of events can become preoccupying activities, as Wendy describes with reference to her husband Roger:

I feel as if I have to try and register, every day your whole life is, when I'm with him I've got to notice things, I've got to notice what he does when he says he doesn't feel well and I've got to try and remember what's happened on a certain day and then leading up to it because when we go to the doctors they need it because he can't tell them, and so you've got to try and take, physically take, you have to take, mentally I mean, take notice of every single silly little thing, or what might seem silly to some people, so that the doctors have got some clue because they're in the same boat as everyone else and its more difficult because I could be guessing wrong, I mean I'm giving this doctor the version of what I see and what I think and I feel sorry for him to be quite honest because I mean its a little bit like a duck treading water and getting nowhere sometimes, and it takes him longer. I said they have to be really really careful as to what they do because they're relying on me and what they can try and understand from Roger, and they could treat him for something he's not got, I said, because we can't explain it properly so its, its a case of going backwards and forwards and when they see a pattern then they can act on it, but they can't before that because its, its really really difficult.

[Question:] Do you feel they [doctors] understand the communication problems?

Yeah they do, they're really kind, they've never ever, I've never felt that we've been a nuisance, never, and that's speaking for the doctor. They, you never feel as if you're a nuisance and when you leave, Dr Martin says, its nice to see you, see you again, and you don't feel, you just don't feel a nuisance and you don't, you don't feel awkward or I don't anyway, I mean we're there and its so frustrating, trying to get to grips with whatever's wrong, but you just don't feel that you, that they're watched in other words, they're not looking at their watches, you don't feel as if they're, they don't make you think well, we've got another patient out there, hurry up and say whatever, we're not getting anywhere and you'd better come back another day. There's none of that, no, they're really good.

Aphasia, time and services

Wendy's point leads to another issue that was constantly raised in both the interview and ethnographic studies: the time pressures on people who deliver health- and social care services to those affected by aphasia. While family members may be willing and able to dedicate time to communication, this is more rarely the case for people working in the caring professions. Talking to institutional carers in residential and nursing homes, the pressures upon them become only too apparent. Often, such workers have to help large numbers of physically frail people to get up, washed and dressed, and finding additional time to dedicate to fathoming out someone's message in the painstaking ways described above is difficult. A nurse working in a residential home, who provided care for a woman with severe aphasia, commented, 'It's unfortunate, but that's the nature of it, we have to think of the mass rather than the individual.'

Talking to therapists in the course of the observation sessions, it became clear that time is also of the essence for professionals working in rehabilitation. One physiotherapist expressed the problem with reference to a person with marked aphasia with whom she was working, as follows:

He just doesn't retain anything and he doesn't do it at home. In here I have got to have motivated patients and I've got to see progress. You can see how busy we are. We had, what was it, seven in this morning. If he doesn't make progress he'll be out after a month. He'll become a review patient, a monitored patient not an on-going patient.

People with aphasia also commented on the timing of the various services they received. Many expressed a desire to have more treatment, more follow-up, and more time with health- and social care practitioners than they actually received. In effect, the ending of services was often not negotiated (another time consuming process) but simply happened: *'They cancelled that. Why, I don't know, but they did. I felt they were wasting their time.'*

Service users and people with aphasia in particular may have a different perspective on the allocation and use of time in the 'therapy session'. Many people who experienced speech and language therapy services, for example, commented on how invaluable they found the one-to-one time spent with the therapist. Harry Clarke, in this volume, corroborates this: 'What she silently gave me though was precious time and space.' While many therapists, like the physiotherapist quoted above, may be focused on that precious therapy time to develop skills and move people on in their recovery, service users refer to protected time away from the outside world, with a skilled listener who might help them understand a little of the turmoil and chaos which has unexpectedly entered their life.

A similar difference in perspective arises in perceptions of time as it relates to the recovery process. Many NHS service providers feel that services extending from between six months to two years after a person's stroke are 'long-term'. In a recent consultation exercise concerning NHS therapy services, a man with aphasia praised the quality and quantity of his speech and language therapy. But he also pointed out that: *'for the first four years I was in a complete fog. I really did not have any idea what my life was or where it was going.'*

This freezing of time in the immediate aftermath of the stroke was frequently mentioned by people with aphasia. Many also described how, as time passes, their aphasia is continuously revealed anew by the changing demands of their social world. This continues years after the onset of aphasia, making the time-span of rehabilitation services seem somewhat limited. One man, who had a stroke when his two boys were very young, found he could cope quite well with talking and reading to them in their early years. Now they are older, the linguistic demands they place upon him have become much more sophisticated. They want him to explain word meanings, how electricity works and so on. This he struggles to do, and has found that his sense of being a good father to them has diminished as a consequence.

People with aphasia deal with the same family troubles and celebrations as everyone else: illness, redundancy, bereavement and divorce, graduation, weddings, the birth of grandchildren. Each of these events places new demands on language and time. It is needed to negotiate services, to say goodbye, to counsel, to make speeches. As time unfolds, aphasia becomes more, not less, apparent. This suggests that conventional timescales for therapy and support may be too restricted, and derived from a short-term view of what aphasia means to those who have it.

Whatever the reason, lack of time often affects the quality of services offered to people with aphasia, in some cases making them effectively inaccessible. Many people with aphasia, while sympathetic to the pressures of work, comment on the poor communication skills of health and social care practitioners, a problem often consolidated by their rushed demeanour:

He is not even taking a time for me. Rush rush rush. I have been frustrated and inside me I feel as if what do I do now?

(Ravi, talking about his general practitioner)

He said: 'Explain what you mean' and of course I couldn't and he sort of sat there tapping his fingers. He said: 'Well does that mean you can't see countryside?'

(Rebecca, an optician, talking about the response of a houseman when she told him her field of vision was disturbed)

Experiences of people who use communication aids (and who therefore take longer to communicate) are not dissimilar. Robillard (1994) writes of his experiences of communicating with a range of healthcare workers in hospital settings. Physicians would request him to prepare what he had to say before their ward rounds but:

this suggestion left out the possibility to respond to any emergent conversation while they were in the room. It also assumed that I would remember what I wanted to say in conversational contexts long after the conversation had passed.

(Robillard 1994: 386)

Robillard also identified how interactions with 'flying nurses' – those at the facility on a short-term contract – were much more difficult than those with 'local authentic nurses'. This second group were people who shared important local social and cultural knowledge. 'There was a reciprocity of highly detailed knowledge which located me and them.' Unlike the flying nurses they were able to follow certain threads of conversation more quickly and demonstrated greater willingness and motivation to attend to Robillard's alphabet board. As Higginbotham and Wilkins (1999) point out, these groups of nurses had both a different perception of the 'fruits to be gained from the time and effort spent in interaction' and a different set of pragmatic resources to draw upon. This point resonates with many of the experiences of people with aphasia, who are exquisitely sensitive to others' levels of investment in interactions with them.

Research is increasingly highlighting how formalized time-frames can create barriers to communication for a wide variety of groups of people when negotiating health and welfare services, and that such temporal restrictions affect the quality of services delivered and received (Warin *et al.* 2000). For example, people whose first language is not English can face problems securing help and advice during doctors' appointments because bureaucratic pressures do not allow enough time for the necessary exchange of information. People with communication impairment are forced by both the formal and informal everyday arrangement of time into unsatisfactory interactions.

It is clear that service users' perspectives on what services should and should not be available differs from what service deliverers have traditionally offered. Thankfully, in the UK and elsewhere, there is now evidence of a genuine commitment to the philosophy of placing patients and the public more authentically at the centre of developing policy and practice (Byng *et al.* 2003). This should reveal the user's concerns for increased time and improvement in time management of services.

Time for inclusion

At Connect we are trying to develop, plan and deliver services in collaboration with people who have aphasia. Numerous consultation exercises have developed the organization's understanding of what inclusion means in practice. In preparing for and carrying out consultation with people who have aphasia, time is a critical resource. Some examples of the extra demands on time include:

- developing accessible materials – marketing the event, supporting materials on the day, aphasia friendly summary documents (for example, attending to clarity of language and using pictures to support understanding of words);
- training and thoroughly briefing group facilitators;
- finding and training sufficient communication supporters to assist with small group discussion;
- working with people with aphasia before, during and after the meeting to support and make the process as efficient as possible;
- allocating sufficient time and sufficient breaks at the meeting which may mean that an event happens over a day or series of meetings rather than in a one-hour meeting;
- allocating sufficient time for thorough rather than superficial debate in the context of aphasia.

Individuals, communities and organizations such as Connect face a steep learning curve as they work towards the genuine inclusion of people with communication impairment. This endeavour is indeed a time consuming business. The need for time is infrastructural, affecting the planning, managing and resourcing of services. It is possible, if challenging, to adapt temporal conventions so that people with diverse styles and paces of communication can be included in the planning and development of accessible services. This perhaps goes some way towards demonstrating how the social and institutional discrimination faced by people living with aphasia can be addressed.

This chapter has focused on how people with aphasia struggle to participate in everyday social interaction and negotiation. People with aphasia have voiced how discrimination faced by disabled people is 'felt' and becomes part of the experience of everyday life through the temporal norms of speech and language use. However, the temporal marginalization and estrangement experienced by people with communication impairment cannot be understood in isolation from the wider material and social status of disabled people as a whole.

The creation of a society that is enabling rather than disabling does not mean accommodating disabled people as an optional extra, it means acting on the basis that their needs and rights are fundamental. Access to services for people with physical and sensory impairments is slowly opening up under increasing pressure from antidiscriminatory legislation. Concrete and spatial barriers seem fairly straightforward both to identify and dismantle, given the political will. Disabling temporal barriers have been less of a priority in antidiscrimination initiatives, perhaps because they are invisible and poorly understood. If temporal barriers are taken seriously their removal has profound implications for the resourcing, planning and organization of services.

Such a recognition is likely to result in a demand for difficult-to-achieve changes in the culture, style and dynamics of personal communication. That said, the inclusion of people who have communication impairments brings many benefits, including the engagement of a skilled and creative force, and less waste and misdirection of resources in the long-term. Time used in this way is well spent.

References

Adam, B. (1995) *Timewatch. The Social Analysis of Time.* Oxford: Polity.

Barnes, C. (1994) *Disabled People in Britain and Discrimination.* London: Hirst & Company.

Boazman, S. (1999) Inside aphasia, in M. Corker and S. French (eds) *Disability Discourse.* Buckingham: Open University Press.

Byng, S., Farrelly, S., Parr, S., Fitzgerald, L. and Ross, S. (2003) *Having a Say: Promoting the Participation of People who have Communication Impairments in Healthcare Decision-making.* London: NHS Health in Partnership Programme.

Corker, M. (1998) *Deaf and Disabled, or Deafness Disabled?* Buckingham: Open University Press.

Corker, M. and French, S. (eds) (1999) *Disability Discourses.* Buckingham: Open University Press.

Finkelstein, V. (1980) *Attitudes and Disabled People: Issues for Discussion.* New York: World Rehabilitation Fund.

French, S. (1992) Equal Opportunities? The Problem of Time, *New Beacon*, 76(1).

Freund, P. (2001) Bodies, disability and spaces: the social model of disabling spatial organisations, *Disability and Society*, 16(5): 689–706.

Gleeson, B. (1999) *Geographies of Disability.* London: Routeldge.

Higginbotham, J. and Wilkins, D. (1999) Slipping through the timestream: social issues of time and timing in augmented interactions, in D. Kovarsky, J. Duchan and M. Maxwell (eds) *Constructing (In)competence: Disabling Evaluations in Clinical and Social Interaction.* Mahwah, NJ: Lawrence Erlbaum.

Imrie, R. (1996) *Disability and the City: International Perspectives.* London: Paul Chapman.

Kagan, A. (1998) Supported conversation for adults with aphasia, *Aphasiology*, 12: 816–30.

Oliver, M. (1983) *Social Work with Disabled People.* London: Macmillan.

Oliver, M. (1990) *The Politics of Disablement*. London: Macmillan.

Parr, S., Byng, S., Gilpin, S. and Ireland, C. (1997) *Talking about Aphasia*. Buckingham: Open University Press.

Parr, S. (2003) *What Happens to People with Severe Aphasia?* Report for the Joseph Rowntree Foundation. London: Joseph Rowntree Foundation.

Paterson, K. (2001) Disability studies and phenomenology: finding a space for both the carnal and the political, in S. Cunningham-Burley and K. Backett-Milburn (eds) *Exploring the Body*. Basingstoke: Palgrave.

Paterson, K. and Hughes, B. (1999) Disability studies and phenomenology: the carnal politics of everyday life, *Disability and Society*, 14(5): 597–610.

Robillard, A.B. (1994) Communication problems in intensive care units, *Qualitative Sociology*, 17: 383–95.

Thompson, E.P. (1974) Time, work-discipline and industrial capitalism, in M.W. Flinn and T.C. Smout (eds) *Essays in Social History*. Oxford: Clarendon Press.

Tregaskis, C. (2002) Social model theory: the story so far, *Disability and Society*, 17(4): 457–70.

UPIAS (1976) *Fundamental Principles of Disability*. London: Union of Physically Impaired Against Segregation.

Wendell, S. (1996) *The Rejected Body. Feminist Philosophical Reflections on Disability*. New York: Routledge.

Zarb, G. (ed.) (1995) *Removing Disabling Barriers*. London: Policy Studies Institute.

Warin, M., Baum, F., Kalucy, E., Murray, C. and Veale, B. (2000) The power of place: space and time in women's and community health centres in South Australia, *Social Science and Medicine*, 50.

Acknowledgements

The two studies of the experience of people with aphasia upon which this chapter draws were funded by the Joseph Rowntree Foundation.

13

Cebrelating aphasia poetry power

Chris Ireland and Carole Pound

Key points

- Chris Ireland is a poet who has aphasia and Carole works with Chris as her 'poetry editor'.
- Chris and Carole have been doing workshops about poetry and aphasia, presenting different poems and talking about people's reactions. In this chapter, Chris presents her poetry in her own words and challenges the audience to think about:
  - language;
  - aphasia;
  - barriers;
  - rebellion;
  - poetry;
  - liberation.
- Some of the poems are about the personal experience of aphasia and some are about disability and the social world.
- Chris and Carole celebrate the language of aphasia by making poetry with aphasia spellings, words and ideas.
- They show the power, creativity and liberation of aphasia language and poetry.

This chapter is based of work, recently years of Chris Ireland and also as Poet-in-Residence at Connect. 'I' – Chris is the poet, thinker, writer. Carole Pound – Director Therapy and Education Connect and 'my main woman', poetry editor, colleague and supporter. We are from two different professional background, pooling expertise.

Also by working with Maria Black, linguist at University College, London. I am indebted to her. We explore of the depth, complexity and creative of aphasia and share about thinking and language challenging to creative richness in work. (See this volume for a chapter written by me and Maria.)

Also I continue working and learning with other people involved with aphasia, friends, life experiences and observations. In working on this work there are many, many drafts, sweat, tears and blood! I need varied scribers, discussion and supporters over the years. Together we share, working and growing together. The chapter probably is demanding and challenging for the readers but hope be accessible for people from varied backgrounds. But as Geoffrey Hill, Poet Professor put it: 'Difficult poetry is the most democrative because you are honouring your audience's intelligence!' Hope you will be interested in the issues in the chapter – or perhaps be challenging – agreeing or disagreeing.

The extract, below, explains about the beginnings:

My language has changed but not how I use it. Like before, I use it to match my feelings, to analyse. I go for meanings, understanding. Language like tools . . . Reading is still hard and less pleasure that before . . . So frustrating: means me cut off to learn knowledge. Belong in my own private word . . . world. Miss reading novels. Catch expression and inner feelings, more like poetry. A big loss. Last evening I tried to read again Lord of the Rings *but I cannot read in the evening. I so weary and ache. I can't follow poetry, understand puns and symbolism. I complain I lost poetry. My friends say I tapped on some new poetry, my own poetry.*

Below is a summary of the elements or themes of aphasia poetry power.

The themes and elements of aphasia poetry power

ACESSIBLE – simplex/complex:
To explore the joy of words/phrases by the route from complex to more available ways. Using visual cues by graphics and auditory cues by music to enhance to appreciate of the poem.

LIBERATOR – personal and collective power as language rebel, personal and more confident. Belonging part of collective VOICE confront to the barriers.

HEALING – new identity and dignity.
Release strong emotions.
Sense of ownership – controlling own language/self respect.

STORYTELLER – 'Communiter'
Communicator/compute/computer/multi parts of varied words which relate together bringing deep thoughts.
Everybody tell their stories – personal stories and social commentary.

PHILOSPHER – observer of life and human issues.
Seeing life/watching around us.
Seeking of meaning of life/universal issues.

CEBRELATION – from double meaning: cebrel- 'thinker/from brain; 'lating' – enlarging pleasure!
Aphasia as a form of art. Creative – seeing and using joy of words.
Using internal rhymth, sounds, pauses and deeper multi-layered understanding.

Since early 1990s, I have to explore about the 'new poetry', to understand more about the personal depth and the social world. So playing and working with language and aphasia to seeking to enjoy and to strive.

Asphasia poetry in motion

There are three versions on the theme of 'asphasia poetry in motion'.
   The first version I presented using by mega media: sound and rhythm by music from opera, Carmen and visual by stills of art of Spanish/Italian countryside and graphics/drawings.
   So imagine by:

- *feeding* your *ears*
- *tasting* your *eyes*
- *treating* your *spirit*
- *touching* your *soul*

ASPHASIA POETRY IN MOTION NUMBER 1

I would love to write opera
I would love to sing opera
I would love to conduct too.
Soul music in me – touch and sense –
Latin favourites
Vivadile, Rossini, Bizet, Puccini
Carmen, Seasons, Dances, Granada

I see music in my head
I touch in my soul – tragedy
I feel in my heart – passion
I am alive again

I so taste Romances
Beeth and Tsch
Beautiful violins
Pulling soul strings

I so hear cello
Elgar and Dvor
Mega – meaconoly
Sounds by Du Pre

I so view Baroke Treasures
Italian landscapes
Soothing my pain

I cannot write concerto
I cannot sing concerto
I cannot conduct too.

But I can find soul language
In Asphasia Poetry in Motion

Inside my own rhymns
Internal rhymn
Sense of separate joys
I cannot really hear it at once
But I can hear them too much
I touch and I feel them
TOO MUCH – TOO MANY . . .
So hope to share with you
So share joy and sad and power
Deep sad – soul power and
Alive joy of internal music.

Before published in the journal, I discussed with the editor. She was correcting. I explained that there are *not* spelling errors but 'creative errors' to show aphasia. Allowed them! Readers were GP/nurses, educating and sharing regarding about the creativity and depth to more understanding of aphasia voice.

But in the second version – I was more careful with 'errors' – because for a wider audience who probably do not know about aphasia. This was in a poetry competition. As an aphasia person, it is very hard and very stressed to put the original version into twenty lines. Indeed, I need help – many conversations and fax with Carole (my poetry 'editor')!

APHASIA POETRY IN MOTION NUMBER 2

I see music in my head
I touch in my soul – tragedy
I feel in my heart – passion.

Taste Romances – Beeth and Tsych –
Beautiful violins – pulling soul strings.
Hear Cello – mega meaconly Elgar and Dvor
Vien Baroke Treasures and Italian landscapes.
Soothing pain and life distress.

Seeking and finding soul language
In Aphasia Poetry in Motion
Inside my own rhymn – Internal rhythm
Sense of separate joys.

I cannot really hear it *at one*
But I can hear them *too much*
I touch and feel them – too much *– too many*
Lost language and at a stroke – aphasia.

In the third version, I enjoyed to explore working on the language. There is more complex – deeper – freer – longer and feeling on *internal rhythm too.*

ASPHASIA POETRY IN MOTION NUMBER 3

Boty/BODY – WREAKED
My heart breaking
Only aching for LOVE . . .
AND UNDERSTANDING
AND CARING AND COMPASSION.
Thank you, Beeth and Tschy . . .
Violins ROMANCES to soothe me
To soothe you too
Thank you VISAUAL LANDSCAPES
TALL TRESS/TREES AND GARRATT GREENS
OUTSIDE of front of home and
OUTSIDE of back of home

Thank for some outside peace
To soothe the aching body and mind
To gift inner peace
To feed soul and spirit
To VOICE the internal rhymn.

To share and voice with
Spring birds and buds and bushes,
Trying to survive in
GLOBAL warming climilate
To calm the inner and outside havoc.
In crazy mega – MOGGY comspol
In the SMOKE to chock/choke us
In the ROAR of monster motors.

ASPHASIA POETRY IN MOTION
NUMBER THREE!!!
Unavailable by demand !!
Too many words in the world
Word – world – wordy – world !!
We own our words and
Pictures for our new world.

Asphasia – asps – asphasia
Own – our – own personal internal rhythm.
Labyrinth spirals to the soul.
In motion – pictures – MUSIC – movement
Touch – smell – feel so deeply
Alive if 'LISTEN TO' !!!

As student and teacher
To share and to understood
TOGETHER
Build up
Compassion, cring world
Lost world and explore word/world and
With asphasia poetry in motion
TO NEW WORD-WORLD!!

Language as a rebel

This is about language as powerful. In losing language there is long and hard struggle and finding ways with support and partnerships to finding your new ways with language.

I look at aphasia as *different* but *not* as deficient.

People tapped on their experiences/backgrounds/professions. I draw from social science/teaching/research (Ireland 1982) community and political activist/counselling (Ireland 1995; Ireland and Wotten 1996).

Also I have always interested language/reading development /psycho-analysis/art and music therapy/enjoy poetry writing/journal/com-plementary therapies.

As cannot able to work, as before, we need to explore new ways to live after loss and find a 'career' or interest but in different ways, involve-ment and continuing growth.

I have always interested in language and emotions. I cannot read novels/newspapers. I cannot do a lot as before the stroke. I concentrate on what I can do – participate in new poetry/creativity, with more rests, breaks and adapting.

This poetry is rooted in writing down/out diaries in private 'raw data' and psychoanalysis including dreams (see Bollas 1991). Also in exploring in articles public (sharing) and lectures, exploring depth of 'errors' in language.

The new poetry is exploring consciously and unconsciously:

- POETRY breaks RULES (consciously);
- APHASIA breaks RULES (unconsciously).

There are many themes: personal and collective issues.

The next poem on language as rebel/language is so powerful shows as challenging and standing up to world as a Liberator. Many times what I *say* might *not match to what I write. There are double – meaning* in aphasia words and depth of meaning. Also try to concentrate on punctuation and timing to guidances to understanding or appreciation.

In analysis it is interesting: make you think about the words/phrases so colour in your message or joy in the picture, making conscious from unconscious.

Poetry use 'coining' (a term-currency to manipulate meaning, con-sciously to use vocabulary for a form of art). Poetry and aphasia, as a medium are challenging to try open and accessible to many people to think and discuss more of deeper feelings and thoughts and universal issues.

LANGUAGE IS REBEL – LANGUAGE IS SO POWERFUL

LANGUAGE is a gift
LANGUAGE is flowing
LANGUAGE is so powerful

More powerful than before
   More scared – more fearful
      More demanding – more exhausting
         More screamful – more scheming
            Not so available and not so understand.

BUT deeper, hidden . . .
Inner and outside . . .
New experiences and new knowledge
Reflect on older experiences
Update knowledge.

INNER LANGUAGE – so busy – so noisy
  OUTER LANGUAGE – so busy – so noisy
    I hope and love
    LANGUAGE BELONE ME!

BEFORE language not belong me
Reflect on older experiences
Found LANGUAGE and then
Lost LANGUAGE at a stroke
BUT with you
FOUND LANGUAGE –
My new language
SO NOW I AM A LANGUAGE REBEL

Still as a language rebel in the next poem, using colour and varying fonts, to bring out, sharing deeper, complex world to become more simplex and accessible. The metaphors/symbols used in the poem are about the personal emotions and daily struggles, bringing out the invisible disability to more visible, more understanding by e.g. 'viel vision' – view/ veil/vie in French and 'crazy mirrors' – reflection of distress. Reminds me of Bollas (1991) a psychoanalysist's study of dreams, poetry invites curiosity 'veiled in enigma' (p.67) 'the veil deceives, it also tantalizes' (p.68).

A$PHASIA
MY   ∧   WORD

My BRAIN is bigger than
My WORDS
Maybe loud cymbols in LIFE.

My WORD is bigger than
My BRAIN
Maybe viel visions insight.

My BLUE is bluer than
My WORLD
Maybe reflect crazy mirrors.

In the PINK more than roseier than
My WAYS
Maybe childlife we lost.

In the RAW more than rawer than
the OTHERS
Maybe body–mind–soul merge in pain.
SPIRALLING down
Hues – rhythm – tingling than
Deeper – **Deeper – DEEPER**
  DEEP at the END.

Analytical VIPERS
INVADE MY SPACE
MAYBE – MY WAYS – MY WORLD –
MY WORD
          A$PHASIA
    MY   ^   **WORD**

After workshops people react in mood and feeling to the poem above:

- 'so right, deeply felt' (an aphasia person);
- 'It feels as if a curtain has lifted . . .';
- 'It's given me insight into the mind of an aphasia person' (a relative);
- '[the poem] seemed to emphasize determination and defiance of the restrictions imposed by aphasia. There's no mistaking the experience behind', 'Maybe "body – mind – soul merge in pain" but we still get a tingle of triumph at the end' (a worker in aphasia field).

Noise barriars

In the book – *Talking about Aphasia* (Parr *et al.* 1997) there are many voices – interviews with 50 people with aphasia. It is very powerful used persons' experiences and their *own* voice.

The book writes about the disabling barriers facing people with aphasia. The summary they face daily are:

ENVIRONMENTAL BARRIARS (physical, e.g. noise, speech and language)
STRUCTURE BARRIARS (resources/services available)
ATTITUDES BARRIARS
INFORMATION BARRIARS (pp. 129/130)

In the foreword of the book I wrote:

This is a collective of voices, often to be listened to and often not heard and often not to understand . . . Each title of each chapter show the flexible, empathetic, powerful medium of language reading and out pick out issues, when the reader ready to.

This book belong to the people who tell their stories . . . living with aphasia is facing daily struggle – pain, confusions, isolating, anxiety – and learning and understanding within the social world so noisy, so stressful, so dirty polluted, needy, greedy . . .

In feedback and empowering people to tell their stories, to filter, open hole the stony wall, graphical strongly powerful. Not only to reflect but also to suggest more clear and helpful advisory support . . . and advocate for invisible disabilities to become more visible.

For aphasia people noise a big barriar. Not only 'noisy environment' outside impede us – hurt us – stop us – stress us to relax/work whatever. But 'NOISE' is as a technical term in language/reading development studies. What invades the person not able to understand – for example, too information/too much background noise/too many words/too much complex syntax/too technical terms. We need ramps in society for people with aphasia.

The next poem about impeding 'noise' as a barrier. Here is playing with language, unconscious/conscious. The term 'barriars' based on thoughts of:

- barricades: hastily erected (defence) ramp across street;
- brair/brier: thorns/friar/fire.

Other metaphors: craggy tracks and goose bellies – onomatopia using particular words/spellings to make the multilayered meanings.

Many are themes in the poem:

- Accessible to aphasia language
- Liberator to control over word-world
- Healing and storyteller to share stories of struggles and barriers
- Philosophy of individual/community to more isolation/more stressful/ and more hostile of social world, less care/more fast . . .

ONLY BARRIARS

BARRIARS across lines-riles
Under – unable to touch
To finger out only
And goosebellies under skin
About . . . what? . . .

SOUNDS across crackling tracks
Out – unable. In my head
Unable to tell
To find word – world only
About . . . what?? . . .

BARRIERS across 'silly – sane – society {uh!}
In only under 'selfish gene'.
Since That – ch – ers – days – ways
To lost community only
About . . . what??? . . .

SOUNDS across mealy misery
In our weary WORLD
Since no time – no care – only scare
To 'ME' culture only
About . . . what??????????

ONLY BARRIARS!!!!!!!!!!!!!!

Again, after the workshops we asked people for their responses:

- 'Everything is a barrier' (an aphasia person);
- 'Bellies – that reminds me of butterflies in the stomach and goose bit of goosebumps' (a relative);
- 'Nice illustration of an alienation which is the inevitable result of the "ME" culture. Emphasises a disillusion that many non-aphasic people will be able to relate to as well. Bringing across a sense of trying to deal with the inner issue of aphasia as well as with the outer issues of an uncaring society . . . I felt a good feeling of anger coming through' (a worker in aphasia field).

In the poetry brings out sense of pride, anger and strength. It fits in the affirmative model of disability:

essentially a non-tragic view of disability and impairment which encompasses positive social identities, both individual and collective, for disabled people grounded in the benefits of lifestyle and life experiences of being impaired and disabled!

(Swain and French 2000: 569)

The poem below, is the first poem using rhyme, very difficult with aphasia. So rhyme and rhymth and tempo, as a rap, limerick, bringing humour, problems in society, hopes. It took a long time, many drafts.

The inspiritation comes from many poets: Benjamin Zephaniah, Wendy Cope, Alice Walker, Lois Keith, Bob Marley (in fact, music and songs are words in rhymth) and even Shakespeare, Chaucer and Dickens!

DRUM RAP
NO – NO – NO – NO –
NOISE A-GRAIN!!

Drumming in my batty – brain,
Slamming in their doory – drain
Base, boring, bumy on their beat,
I no – know moaning on my seat.

No – No – No – No NOISE, A-GRAIN!!

Swimming in my gutty – tum,
Laughing in their cruel – gum.
Not toot, now *blairr,* now *nasty,*
Monsters, dirt and loud greedy.

No – No – No – No NOISE, A-GRAIN!!

Popping pills they dole – ing out,
Stopping us to ask about,
Problems but desk dragon – fly
Barriers to puff demon – pie

No – No – No – No NOISE, A GRAIN !!

Stranding a – gain, how get home,
Filling a – nxis, a – no ther form,
Hate phone, mixed messages,
Taxi not come, silly sausages.

No – No – No – No NOISE, A GRAIN !!

Bottling up and so distressed,
Screaming out, so expressed.
No woman – no cry – they say,
Why not – grumble, moan some day!?

No – No – No – No NOISE, A GRAIN !!

Challenging trenched governments
Lessing busy confusements.
So please – no more – no more din,
Stop hitting out in our chin.
No – No – No – No NOISE, A GRAIN !!

Soothing rhythm – gentle rap,
Spiriting – soul, dancing tap.
More partner conversations
Open to REAL communications.
No – No – No – No NOISE, A GRAIN !!

So people – no cry – dry tears
Eased our community fears.
Sell social isolation,
Party – poem celebration.

Yes – Yes – Yes – Yes YEAST of LIFE!!

Sound bites!

After *noise* we more on to sounds with bites! Next poem is 'S-S-S-S-S-S-S- Six (nonsense) Sounds (of Aphasia)!' The question is are they 'nonsense' words?

What is nonsense or not? The roots or reason behind words? Analyse, if appropriate, but careful not over analyse.

This poem relate personal thoughts/experience:

1 The first time I went to a speech/language therapist was when I was six. The school sent me. My mother was very embarrassed ('What is wrong about my daughter's language'?) The therapist give practice on 's' – because a lisp. I felt there was a problem with my language. As a child I was nervous to use words with 's'. So the poem is about playing practise on 's'!!

2 Another experience – a teacher puts us down in our language, saying: 'Middlesborough accent is the *most ugly* in the world!!' She tried to get rid our accent. (Now obvious it doesn't worked on me!!) But I lost lot of confidence as a Northern to come to university in London and made me scared to open my mouth in seminars.

   But this experience resolved me to explore, not only to explore social scientist issues, but also working with young people with language issues and awareness and confident building.

3 After the stroke, I was back with speech/language therapy. Some

researchers wanted to look at some – different words listing on computer, with heavy head phones to make quick responses. Hard work! So the poem below is to get back to them!

In action, in lectures, the speech therapist students were invited to perform! One person were asked each different silly sound and vary music mood to introduce each verse. Also graphic images are used to signpost to help understanding.

Some students from City University, helped with typing graphics and preparing some poems for workshops to present at Connect. Hope helps them in their understanding and they helped with more accessibility for people with aphasia.

S – S – S – S – S – S
SIX NONSENSE SOUNDS (of Asphasia)

I love Ssi - - - - Silly SOUNDS
Grup – blump – pissy
Mussy – luppy – TWITY
Niss – Tsychi – silly
NONSENSE *sounds? ! ?*

As speech/language therapist research
Why they like Ssi - - - - silly Sounds
(of Asphasia)?

I touch Ssa ——— sad SOUNDS
Blue – bluey – bluest
Bummy – bump – Blump
BUM *– blast – Bluggest*
Nonsense *sounds?!?*
As word – world poverty and tragedy
Why we need to Ssa - - - - Sad Sounds
(of Asphasia)?

I have SSh _____ shitty SOUNDS
Fech – foggy – fluest
He/r – forei – sh-shore
Sheerr – STROKE – surgest
Nonsense *sounds?!?*
As so much pain and ill – NOISE in life
Why there is so much SSh _____ shitty Sounds
(of Asphasia)?

I need Sso _____ soothing SOUNDS
Sooothe – sheer – shore
Seea – sand – RIPPLEY
Touchy – gentleey – warmrthe
Nonsense *sounds ?!?*
As so deparsate need for gentle CARE
Why not everyone for Sso _____ soothing Sounds

(of Asphasia)

I reach Sse _____ sensual SOUNDS
Sensses – senslee – sexxy
Touchy – luvy – nippley
Knoby – OH OH *– shoky*
Nonsense *sounds?!?*
As dody – body merging together
Why not *healing for Sse _____ sensual Sounds*

(of Asphasia)

I want Ssu _____ survival SOUNDS
Strrong – gong – hopes
Culturee – gangy – withit
Ancest – partee – GUTTS!
Nonesense *sounds?!?*
As Knack – asphasia need to hear us!
Why not 'RIGHT OUT' *for*
    Ssu _____ SURVIVAL SOUNDS

(of Asphasia)?

Hope you enjoyed the sounds and guessing what could they be!

Aphasia poetry can be a vehicle, as an education inside to out or out to inside and as a form of art. An example is to explain in an extract from the poem hero Workshirt or Stroke Villians:

HERO WORKSHIRT OR STROKE VILLIANS

So inspire by perspire or exspire!
At the STROKE – Epochs and Elipse and Epics!
So we need a good listening to and
Really to be HEARD – REALLY TO BE HEARD,
As by power – People Flush Overflowed.

Bolton (1999) writes about the therapy of potential of creative writing and discusses about the healing and power in varied writing processes. Also Hunt and Sampson (1998) examine about the theory and practice of creative writing as a therapeutic tool. The question is about how to enable people with aphasia in creative writing? We are beginning in the exploration in the presentations, workshops and discussions at Connect. Also hope accessible for non-aphasia people too! – inside out and outer in – a form of art for all!

In this chapter, people with aphasia are viewed as a minority group: As other minority groups in Britain, for example, older, disabled, ill, poor, unemployed, homeless and some ethnic groups are as dispossessed or invisibility or not understood. As other minority groups across the world, for example, Aboriginal/Maori/Native American post-colonized countries: in Africa/South America/India. As one of various form of art are used to fight back, belonging in a creativity community – richness in soul and energy in spirit – art poetry protest!

Aphasia, as foreign in ones language, as a language minority group, colonized by some kind of brain invading insult and often prejudized/ discriminated in society. An invisible group has little power, few resources and often isolated. So we need strong allies! (see Pound *et al.* 2000).

Endings–beginnings–doing!

In concluding, I hope all of us can work to a 'language of humanity' across the world by each of us with 'little deeds – ways'. For many, people with aphasia, relatives and friends, medicals, therapists, public etc. often see aphasia as a problem – demanding and difficult. The chapter does not denied that aphasia brings struggles and pain. But hope that the poems and thoughts and experiences demonstrate bringing the richness and 'cebrelating' of the differences and diversity in aphasia and in life and in the word-world!

INSIDE OUT

Washing my mind thoughts
—ripple—ripple—still—still
Balming sounds worms waves in head
—light thro' prism to rainbow spectum
Catch web-dreams words on lint paper
—gentle toasty-taste whisper
*   touch paper, as torch paper!*

Mingling yours' desire, pleasure, polish,
With put mines' passon, creative, rebel,
Together almonds-reminds of hopes of larger picture
Of joy, thinking on to myself precious diamonds – dial-logs,
Picture windows of wind-chimes, windmills

Sails of feel mind in – move-ment
   free mind, as mindfield!

As London Rainforest Gardens,
Drops of chil-call early morning mist,
As jewels of bird songs sing, fresh
—of coal-cool air, saviour-savour,
—of BEING reflective pools, deep echoes,
—of shared work-world-word earth
—of small world dreaming-drumming
—of rhymn in full tasteful-tactive
—of unexpected guests-flowers of plum–cherry
or gnats-bats-rats from hell
To excite to creative leaps of gutright
   planes and trains to INSIDE OUT!!

Bibliography

Black, M. and Ireland, C. (2002) Talking to ourselves: Dialogues in and out of language. This volume.

Bollas, C. (1991) *The Shadow of the Object – Psychoanalysis of the Unthought Known*. London: Free Association Books.

Bolton, G. (1999) *The Therapeutic Potential of Creative Writing*. London: Jessica Kingsley.

Campo, R. (1997) *The Poetry of Healing*. London: W.W. Norton & Comp.

Hunt, C. and Sampson, F. (1998) *The Self on the Page*. London: Jessica Kingsley.

Ireland, C. and Black, M. (1992) Living with aphasia: the insight story, *UCL Working Paper in Linguistics*, 4.

Ireland, C. (1982) Talking in class – language and learning, in the Vauxhall Papers, *Becoming Our Own Experts*, Talk Workshop Group. London: Redwood Burn.

Ireland, C.M. (1995) 100 years on from Freud's *On Aphasia*: from patient to counsellor, in C. Code and D. Muller (eds) *Treatment of Aphasia: From Theory to Practice*. London: Whurr Publishers.

Ireland, C. and Wotten, G. (1996) Time to talk: counselling for people with dysphasia, *Disability and Rehabilitation*, 11: 585–9.

Pound, C., Parr, S. Lindsay, J. and Woolf, C. (2000) *Beyond Aphasia: Therapies for Living with Communication Disability*. Bicester: Speechmark.

Parr S., Byng, S. and Gilpin, S. with Ireland, C. (1997) *Talking About Aphasia*. Buckingham: Open University Press.

Swain, J. and French, S. (2000) Towards an affirmation model of disability, *Disability and Society*, 14(4): 569–82.

Acknowledgements

Particular I am appreciated of Claire Wills and Jane de la Haye. There are other acknowledgements and thanks to colleagues and friends: Judy Duchan, Susie Parr, Sally Byng, David Bennett, Sally Inman, Sue Boazman, Hugh Hansell, Teresa Regan, Hazel Macauley, Heather and Jim McNally, Angela Sizer, and some students from City University.

Index

TALKING ABOUT APHASIA

Susie Parr, Sally Byng and Sue Gilpin with Chris Ireland

> What is aphasia actually like – for those who have lost language, and those around them? What impact does it have on people's lives? Can the fearful communication gap somehow be bridged? Here is a book which addresses these questions and innumerable other related issues, with the most meticulous research and the most accessible descriptions. *Talking About Aphasia* will be equally valuable for professionals and patients alike, as well as the families, friends and therapists of those with aphasia.
>
> Oliver Sacks

> This book is a wonderful idea and it meets a heretofore unmet need. It derives from a particularly interesting database, since it deals with aphasia in aphasic people's own language . . . It is strongly recommended.
>
> Professor Audrey Holland, Department of Speech Pathology,
University of Arizona, USA

This book is about living with aphasia – a language impairment which can result from stroke. Drawing on in-depth interviews with fifty aphasic people, it explores the experience of aphasia from the dramatic onset of stroke and loss of language to the gradual revelation of its long-term consequences. The story is told from the perspective of aphasic people themselves. They describe the impact of aphasia upon their employment, education, leisure activities, finances, personal relationships and identity. They describe their changing needs and how well these have been met by health, social care and other services. They talk about what aphasia means to them, the barriers encountered in everyday life and how they cope. The book offers a unique insight into the struggle of living with aphasia, combining startlingly unusual language with a clear interlinking text.

Contents

What is aphasia? – 'Is frightened. Is frightened': the early experience of stroke and aphasia – 'The thing is – what job?': work, leisure and aphasia – Can I get a word in edgeways?': family friends and aphasia – 'Lost in the undertow': health, social care and voluntary services for people with aphasia – 'Everything seems a secret': information and aphasia – 'Doing the inside work': the meaning of aphasia – 'They cannot see it so how will they know?'; aphasia and disability – 'I'm fed up of saying I'm sorry': learning to live with aphasia – Appendix: about the project – Further reading.

160pp   0 335 19936 4 (Paperback)   0 335 19937 2 (Hardback)

CONTROVERSIAL ISSUES IN A DISABLING SOCIETY

John Swain, Sally French and Colin Cameron

At its best Disability Studies is an arena of critical debate addressing controversial issues concerning not just the meaning of disability but the nature of society, dominant values, quality of life, and even the right to live. Indeed, Disability Studies is itself the subject of controversy, in terms of its theoretical basis and who controls courses and research and whether it should be shaped and controlled by disabled academics or grassroots activists. Within these debates, generated by the social model of disability, are fundamental challenges to policy, provision and professional practice that are directly relevant to all who work with disabled people, whether in the field of social work, health or education.

Controversial Issues in a Disabling Society has been written specifically to raise questions and stimulate debate. It has been designed for use with students in group discussion, and to support in-depth study on a variety of professional courses. It covers a wide range of specific, substantive issues within Disability Studies in a series of succinct chapters. Each chapter sets a question for debate, places the key issues in context and presents a particular argument. This is an accessible and engaging book which challenges dominant positions and ideologies from a social model viewpoint of disability.

Contents

c.192pp   0 335 20904 1 (Paperback)   0 335 20905 X (Hardback)

GENDER AND AGEING
CHANGING ROLES AND RELATIONSHIPS

Sara Arber, Kate Davidson and Jay Ginn (Eds.)

This book is a follow-up to Arber and Ginn's award winning *Connecting Gender and Ageing* (1995). It contains original chapters from eminent writers on gender and ageing, addressing newly emergent areas within gender and ageing, including gender identity and masculinity in later life.

Early work on gender and ageing was dominated by a focus on older women. The present collection breaks with this tradition by emphasizing changing gender roles and relationships, gender identity and an examination of masculinities in midlife and later life. A theme running through the book is the need to reconceptualize partnership status, in order to understand the implications of both widowhood and divorce for older women and men, as well as new forms of relationships, such as Living Apart Together (LAT-relationships). There is also an underlying focus on how socio-economic circumstances influence the experiences of ageing and the ways transitions are negotiated.

Written with undergraduate students and researchers in mind, *Gender and Ageing* will be an invaluable text for those studying social gerontology, sociology of later life, gender studies, health and community care and social policy.

Contents

Changing approaches to gender and later life – Theorizing gender and age relations: what of men and masculinities? – Changing perspectives on age, gender and life after work – Reconceptualizing intimacy and ageing: living apart together – Sex and ageing: a gendered issue – Bringing outsiders in: gay and lesbian family ties over the life course – Reconceptualizing gender and partnership status: integrating socio-economic position and social involvement – Gender, partnership status and pension poverty – Getting by without a spouse: living arrangements and support of older people in Italy and Britain – Social networks and social well-being of older men and women living alone – Exploring the social worlds and health behaviours of older men – Sleep as a social act: a window onto gender roles and relationships – Reconceptualizing gender and ageing: drawing the threads together – Index.

192pp   0335 21319 7 (Paperback)   0335 21320 0 (Hardback)

PARTNERSHIPS IN FAMILY CARE

Mike Nolan, Ulla Lundh, Gordon Grant and John Keady (Eds.)

- What are the key features of partnerships between family and professional carers?
- How do partnerships change over time?
- What is needed to help create the best working partnerships?

Forging partnerships between service users, family carers and service providers is a key theme in both the policy and academic literatures. However, what such partnerships mean and how they can be created and sustained while responding to change over time, is far from clear.

This book considers how family and professional carers can work together more effectively in order to provide the highest quality of care to people who need support in order to remain in their own homes. It adopts a temporal perspective looking at key transitions in caregiving and suggests the most appropriate types of help at particular points in time. It draws on both empirical and theoretical sources emerging from several countries and relating to a number of differing caregiving contexts in order to illustrate the essential elements of 'relationship-centred' care.

Partnerships in Family Care will be important reading for all health care students and professionals with an interest in community and home care for the ill, disabled, and elderly.

Contents
Preface – Introduction: Why another book on family care? – Part One: 'Recognizing the need' and 'taking it on' – The dynamics of dementia – Early interventions in dementia: carer-led evaluations – Seeking partnerships between family and professional carers – Part Two: Working through it – Quality care for people with dementia – Partnerships with families over the life course – 'I wasn't aware of that' – Caring for people with dementia – Family care decision-making in later life – Part Three: 'Reaching the end' and 'a new beginning' – The evolving informal support networks of older adults with learning disability – Relatives' experiences of nursing home entry – Placing a spouse in a care home for older people – Creating community – Forging partnerships in care homes – Conclusion: New Directions for partnerships relationship-centred care – References – Index.

Contributors
Christine Bigby, Louise Brereton, Denise Chaston, Chris Clark, Sue Davies, Irene Ericson, Gordon Grant, Ingrid Hellstrom, Prue Ingram, John Keady, Gwynnyth Llewellyn, Ulla Lundh, Rhonda Nay, Mike Nolan, Asa Paulsson, Alan Pearson, Jonas Sandberg, Bev Taylor, Roger Watson, Bridget Whittell.

320pp   0 335 21261 1 (Paperback)   0 335 21262 X (Hardback)

SOCIAL THEORY, SOCIAL POLICY AND AGEING
A CRITICAL INTRODUCTION

Carroll Estes, Simon Biggs and Chris Phillipson

In this important new book, three leading social theorists of old age present a critical review of key theoretical developments and issues influencing the study of adult ageing. The authors explore contemporary trends in social policy drawing on the experience of ageing in the USA, Europe and an increasingly global environment.

Particular attention is given to feminist perspectives on ageing, ethics and bio-medicine, successful and productive ageing, globalization and migration and the politics of ageing. Consideration is given in each case to the interaction between structural influences on social ageing and the experience of age and identity. The work ends with a manifesto for social theory, social policy and social change.

Social Theory, Social Policy and Ageing will be valuable reading for advanced students and practitioners taking courses in social theory, the sociology of old age and social gerontology.

Contents

0 335 20906 8 (Paperback)   0 335 20907 6 (Hardback)

openup
ideas and understanding
in social science

www.**openup**.co.uk

 **Browse, search and
order online**

 **Download detailed
title information and
sample chapters***

*for selected titles

www.**openup**.co.uk